CONE BEAM COMPUTED TOMOGRAPHY

A Clinician's Guide to 3D Imaging

CONE BEAM COMPUTED TOMOGRAPHY

A Clinician's Guide to 3D Imaging

Prashant P Jaju MDS
Associate Professor
Department of Oral Medicine and Radiology
Rishiraj College of Dental Sciences and Research Centre
Bhopal, Madhya Pradesh, India

Foreword

Stuart C White

JAYPEE The Health Sciences Publisher
New Delhi | London | Philadelphia | Panama

Jaypee Brothers Medical Publishers (P) Ltd

Headquarters

Jaypee Brothers Medical Publishers (P) Ltd
4838/24, Ansari Road, Daryaganj
New Delhi 110 002, India
Phone: +91-11-43574357
Fax: +91-11-43574314
Email: jaypee@jaypeebrothers.com

Overseas Offices

J.P. Medical Ltd
83 Victoria Street, London
SW1H 0HW (UK)
Phone: +44 20 3170 8910
Fax: +44 (0)20 3008 6180
Email: info@jpmedpub.com

Jaypee-Highlights Medical Publishers Inc
City of Knowledge, Bld. 237, Clayton
Panama City, Panama
Phone: +1 507-301-0496
Fax: +1 507-301-0499
Email: cservice@jphmedical.com

Jaypee Medical Inc.
The Bourse
111 South Independence Mall East
Suite 835, Philadelphia, PA 19106, USA
Phone: +1 267-519-9789
Email: jpmed.us@gmail.com

Jaypee Brothers Medical Publishers (P) Ltd
17/1-B Babar Road, Block-B, Shaymali
Mohammadpur, Dhaka-1207
Bangladesh
Mobile: +08801912003485
Email: jaypeedhaka@gmail.com

Jaypee Brothers Medical Publishers (P) Ltd
Bhotahity, Kathmandu, Nepal
Phone: +977-9741283608
Email: kathmandu@jaypeebrothers.com

Website: www.jaypeebrothers.com
Website: www.jaypeedigital.com

Inquiries for bulk sales may be solicited at: jaypee@jaypeebrothers.com

Cone Beam Computed Tomography: A Clinician's Guide to 3D Imaging

First Edition: **2015**

ISBN 978-93-5152-639-1

Printed at Ajanta Offset & Packagings Ltd., New Delhi

Dedicated to

Diya and Mayank

Contributors

Avani Dixit Gandhi MDS
Associate Professor and Guide
Department of Oral Medicine and Radiology
Swami Devi Dyal Dental College and Hospital
Panchkula, Haryana, India
Role of Cone Beam Computed Tomography in Orthodontics and Airway Analysis

Prashant P Jaju MDS
Associate Professor
Department of Oral Medicine and Radiology
Rishiraj College of Dental Sciences and Research Centre
Bhopal, Madhya Pradesh, India
Cone Beam Computed Tomography: Physics and Artifacts
Role of Cone Beam Computed Tomography in Prosthodontics
Role of Cone Beam Computed Tomography in Oral and Maxillofacial Pathologies
Future of Cone Beam Computed Tomography
Limitations of Cone Beam Computed Tomography

Prashant V Suvarna MDS
Professor
Department of Oral Medicine and Radiology
People's College of Dental Sciences and Research Centre
Bhopal, Madhya Pradesh, India
Need of Cone Beam Computed Tomography in Dentistry

Pratik Dedhia MDS
Associate Professor
Department of Oral Medicine and Radiology
Terna Dental College
Navi Mumbai, Maharashtra, India
Role of Cone Beam Computed Tomography in Periodontal Disease

Sushma P Jaju MDS
Assistant Professor
Department of Operative Dentistry and Endodontics
Rishiraj College of Dental Sciences and Research Centre
Bhopal, Madhya Pradesh, India
History of Cone Beam Computed Tomography
Anatomical Landmarks on Cone Beam Computed Tomography
Role of Cone Beam Computed Tomography in Prosthodontics
Role of Cone Beam Computed Tomography in Endodontics and Caries Diagnosis
Role of Cone Beam Computed Tomography in Forensic Odontology

Yoshinori Arai DDS PhD
Nihon University School of Dentistry
1-8-13 Kanda-Surugadai
Chiyoda-ku, Tokyo, Japan
Future of Cone Beam Computed Tomography

Contributors for Photographs

Alessandro Motroni MS (Biomedical Engineer)
Technical Manager
3diemme Sri via Risorgimento
922063 Cantu (Co), Italy
Future of Cone Beam Computed Tomography (Figs 10.2, 10.3, 10.4)

Ashish Mittal BDS MBA PGDM
General Manager
Sirona Dental System Pvt Ltd
Mumbai, Maharashtra, India
Cone Beam Computed Tomography: Physics and Artifacts (Figs 2.3A and B)
Anatomical Landmarks on Cone Beam Computed Tomography (Fig. 4.43)
Role of Cone Beam Computed Tomography in Orthodontics and Airway Analysis (Figs 6.13 and 6.14)
Role of Cone Beam Computed Tomography in Endodontics and Caries Diagnosis (Fig. 7.1)
Role of Cone Beam Computed Tomography in Oral and Maxillofacial Pathologies (Figs 8.1 and 8.18)

Beatriz Gomez Bonilla MDS
Oral Maxillofacial Radiologist
Begmax Radiology Centre
Santiago, Chile
Role of Cone Beam Computed Tomography in Oral and Maxillofacial Pathologies (Figs 8.7, 8.8A to E, 8.10A to D, 8.11A and B, 8.12, 8.16A and B)

Maha Eshaq MDS
Department of Oral and Maxillofacial Radiology
Faculty of Oral and Dental Medicine
Minia University Minya, Egypt
Role of Cone Beam Computed Tomography in Oral and Maxillofacial Pathologies (Figs 8.21A to D, 8.22A and B, 8.23A to D, 8.24A and B, 8.25A to D)

Niranjan Vatkar MDS
Senior Lecturer
Department of Operative Dentistry and Endodontics
MA Rangoonwala Dental College and Hospital
Pune, Maharashtra, India
Role of Cone Beam Computed Tomography in Endodontics and Caries Diagnosis (Figs 7.2 A to D, 7.3A to D)

Praveen B MDS
Oral Maxillofacial Surgery
Private Practitioner
Chennai, Tamil Nadu, India
Role of Cone Beam Computed Tomography in Orthodontics and Airway Analysis (Figs 6.11A to D, 6.12A to C)

Shikha Rathi Diplomate
Consultant, Private Practice
American Board of Oral and Maxillofacial Radiology
Houston, Texas, Southern United States
Anatomical Landmarks on Cone Beam Computed Tomography (Figs 4.16, 4.17, 4.19, 4.26, 4.27, 4.28, 4.29, 4.30, 4.31, 4.44, 4.46, 4.47, 4.48, 4.49, 4.53)
Role of Cone Beam Computed Tomography in Oral and Maxillofacial Pathologies (Figs 8.19, 8.20)

Technodent JSD
CBCT Diagnostic Centre
Bengaluru, Karnataka, India
Role of Cone Beam Computed Tomography in Oral and Maxillofacial Pathologies (Figs 8.13A to C, 8.14A to E)

Foreword

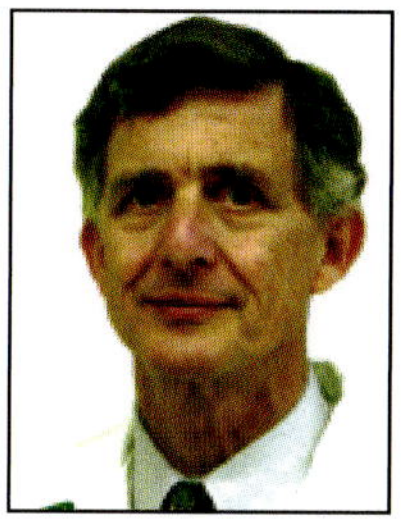

Cone beam imaging, now in its second decade of use in dentistry, has a profound and positive impact on patient care. Clinical experience and systematic investigations have shown its value in detecting disease as well as monitoring disease progression or healing. For varied conditions, such as periapical lesions, impactions, cysts and tumors, sinus disease, fractures, lesions of the temporomandibular joint (TMJ), and many others, cone beam computed tomography (CBCT) offers many diagnostic advantages compared to conventional imaging. This technology is here to stay and will improve in future.

Just with the use of any examination involving ionizing radiation, the dentist must consider the justification for using CBCT imaging. It is important to have a clear understanding of the comparative capabilities and limitations of CBCT and other conventional imaging, to identify those situations where there is a reasonable expectation that a CBCT examination will offer clinically useful information not available with conventional imaging. Limiting the use of CBCT imaging to these situations will reduce unnecessary patient exposure, loss of professional time and expenditure of scarce health-care resources.

When a patient's clinical indications justify the need for CBCT imaging, the dentist will want to optimize the use of this technology. By optimizing the CBCT examination, the patient will be spared from unnecessary exposure and the dentist will maximize the opportunities to obtain the diagnostic information from the examination. This book describes various means to improve the imaging technique including when to limit the field of view, both to reduce patient exposure and to improve image contrast. It is equally important to learn how to optimize the image to improve interpretation? This book provides many illustrations of how to best the orient image slices for a particular patient and diagnostic problem, how to use all three orthogonal image planes, how to vary image brightness and contrast to visualize various features of a lesion, and how to recognize image artifacts. It is important that the user of this technology becomes intimately familiar with the various display options of their image display software. Cross-sectional imaging, surface renderings, maximum intensity imaging, and other display modes all have important roles in visualizing disease and abnormalities.

The importance of systematically reading the entire image volume cannot be stressed. In my personal experience I have seen several instances where seemingly simple cases, such as making measurements in an alveolar ridge for a planned implant placement, became far more complex when systematic review of all the images revealed previously unsuspected tumors. All examinations should be thoroughly reviewed in all three planes, from top-to-bottom, front-to-back or side-to-side, and the findings reported in the patient's record. If a dentist is uncomfortable with the complex anatomy beyond the alveolar ridges or the radiographic manifestations of infections, cysts, tumors and other conditions, I urge them to use the services of an oral radiology individuals trained in this field.

This book will help dentists to learn how to recognize situations where CBCT imaging is indicated, and how to optimize the examination and interpretation of the resulting images. Please read the book and learn its lessons. You and your patients will be the better off as a result.

Stuart C White MDS
Distinguished Professor Emeritus
Department of Oral and Maxillofacial Radiology
UCLA School of Dentistry
Los Angeles, California, USA

Preface

As dentistry evolves within the digital age, manufacturers develop and introduce, but oral healthcare professionals continue to incorporate technological innovations to enhance their practice, as well as improve predictability and productivity of day-to-day dental operations, especially dental implantology with prosthetic restoration of missing teeth. A decade age the first cone beam computed tomography (CBCT) system, the NewTom (QR Inc, Verona, Italy now a Cefla company), received patent approval in Europe. That system required the patient to be placed supine, and in appearance it mimicked fan-beam CT scanners used in medicine. The NewTom provided a low dose, reasonably affordable 3D radiograph imaging system for use in the dental office. To that point, the 3D in imaging had usually meant either blurry or magnified film-based linear tomograms or referral to a medical radiology office, where the CT system was focused at the whole body rather than the maxillofacial region, and the operators were not always cognizant of the diagnostic needs of dentists or the relatively high radiation exposure to the patient. Dental CT can be performed either by CBCT or by multislice CT, but the latter generally results in substantially higher doses to the patient.

Now the CBCT systems are abound, both in numbers and variety, and are already quite common in dental practices and dental imaging centers throughout the world; they are supine systems (e.g. Cefla/QR NewTom 3G, Cefla/Myray SkyView), sit down systems (e.g. ISI/i-CAT, Gendex CB500, ISI/Soredex SCANORA 3D, J Morita Accuitomo, PreXion 3D, 3M ILUMA Elite) and stand-up units (e.g. Cefla/NewTom VG, J Morita Veraviewepocs 3D, Kodak 9000 and 9500, E-Woo/Vatech Picasso Trio, Suni 3D, Sirona Galileos). There are large field of view (FOV) systems that can be used in evaluating craniofacial anomalies and planning orthognathic surgery, where multislice CT would have been used previously, at much higher radiation dosages to the patient. Generally, such as full FOV systems are employed at relatively low-isotropic voxel resolution (i.e. 0.2–0.4 mm) to reduce the dose needed, while reducing image noise and also to permit reasonable reconstruction times.

At the other end of the spectrum, there are small FOV systems that usually provide higher resolution (i.e. often 0.1 mm isotropic voxel resolution or better) that are ideal for such situations as endodontic assessments. These small FOV systems may be hybrid, providing 2D digital panoramic and/or cephalograms (e.g. Orthophos XG 3D, Sirona Germany, Kodak 9000 3D, Carestream). Small FOV systems can provide limited (i.e. 'focused field') volume images of several teeth for approximately the same dose as two traditional intraoral radiographs. Given that such multiple traditional images at different angles could be needed to evaluate an endodontic problem, small FOV CBCT might actually result in a dose savings to the patient.

The CBCT is an adjunct to 2D imaging in dentistry. The 3D imaging provides a clear relationship between structures that could be obscure on 2D images. The CBCT is useful for assessing impacted teeth, particularly the relationship between mandibular third molars and mandibular canals. It is also valuable in assessing implant positioning and preimplant bone augmentation to provide the best possible prosthodontics reconstructive outcome.

Small FOV CBCT is valuable in assessing failed endodontics and perhaps also in primary evaluation of certain teeth prior to endodontics. However, CBCT does not replace 2D imaging of dental caries. Beam hardening artifact from restorations and tooth enamel would result in a very large number of false positives for dental caries, for which current CBCT systems should be used for caries detection.

While the recent graduates from dental school may have some grounding in 3D imaging and direct experience with CBCT during their studies, this varies between institutions. Most dentists already in practice have limited or no training in using 3D images for dental practice and there are a few existing pointers for optimizing CBCT patient image selection. For this reason, this book is particularly useful for demonstrating the value of 3D imaging for the specific purpose of dental implant planning.

The 3D imaging provides accurate anatomic relationships between structures and is much easier to explain (often with simulations) to the patient. One might not always be able to preserve the integrity of the mandibular canal when extracting a third molar, even given a 3D image, but one is more aware of potential complications and best approaches. The patient also is better informed before consenting to the procedure.

There might be practitioners who have relied upon panoramic images to place dental implants for three decades or more, and these 'gurus' often do not see any need to move from what they perceive to be success, until they experience 3D images and see where they were actually placing the implants previously! After that enlightenment, 3D imaging becomes the rule. One can teach an 'old dentist' new tricks, at least when it comes to dental implantology. This is a benefit for both the dentist and the patient.

This book highlights the importance of CBCT in dentistry and its possible future applications in the allied fields.

Prashant P Jaju
E-mail: docprashantjaju@gmail.com

Acknowledgments

Cone beam computed tomography (CBCT) has revolutionized dental practice and now created a virtual 3D world in all aspects of clinical dentistry. It was my dream to share my experience of CBCT with the help of this book.

The book of this magnitude is possible only due to assistance and support from a considerable number of people. I am grateful to the pioneers of dental imaging, in particular its utilization in implant imaging. I owe an enormous debt to the gifted oral radiologists of this age, who seek to expand the envelope of their knowledge. They are my real contributors. The book is a culmination of many years of contemplating fundamental principles conveyed by early researchers, continually scrutinizing the literature to remain abreast of advances and refining illustrative material.

First and foremost, I wish to acknowledge the work of our esteem contributors for their enormous efforts, which is highly appreciated. I feel privileged to have the opportunity to work closely with such talented people. Particular acknowledgment is extended to Professor Emeritus, Dr Stuart C White and President of AAOMR and Dr Allan Farman, for extending their sea of knowledge towards this textbook. Both the legendary oral radiologists had no apprehension in contributing towards this book.

I also wish to thank Dr Yoshinori Arai, who has given insight on the future of CBCT in dentistry.

Younger oral radiologists in the form of Dr Shikha Rathi and Dr Beatriz Gomez, have been kind enough to share their work and experience in this venture. I am also grateful and feel indebted towards Dr John Ludlow, Nerijus Sukaitis, who allowed to reprint their work in our book.

Radiology book requires good quality images, these were provided by dear friends, Dr B Praveen, Dr Niranjan Vatkar, Dr Maha Eshaq, Mr Jayakumar (Technodent JSD).

A special mention of Dr Ashish Mittal, General Manager Sirona India and Sirona team, Germany, who unselfishly allowed us to publish their recent advances in this book.

I also wish to express my sincere thanks to Mr Alessandro Motroni, who allowed us to use the third party software images.

I also wish to extend my gratitude towards the management of our respective colleges without whom this book would have not become a reality. This textbook would not have been completed without the timely, valuable, knowledgeable and enthusiastic contributions of my teacher and guide, Dr Rajiv Desai and Dr Vaibhav Avinashe.

I also take this opportunity to express my gratitude towards my core team, Dr Prashant P Suvarna, Dr Avani Dixit Gandhi, Dr Pratik Dedhia and my beloved wife Dr Sushma P Jaju, who have worked tirelessly to make this book a success. Special mention of my wife Sushma, who was the brain behind designing and compiling of this work. Finally, I wish to thank my family and son Mayank, for their unwavering love, encouragement and moral support not only made my life; easier, but was ultimately the most important force ensuring a successful result.

This is not merely a book of experiences with CBCT, but a combined effort of all of the above. Through their efforts, I hope that I have been able to describe the state of CBCT in present era.

Finally, I thank Shri Jitendar P Vij (Group Chairman), Mr Ankit Vij (Group President), Mr Tarun Duneja (Director–Publishing) and all staff of Bengaluru branch of M/s Jaypee Brothers Medical Publishers (P) Ltd, New Delhi, India, for their encouragement and support, which made this book possible.

Contents

1

Chapter

History of Cone Beam Computed Tomography

Sushma P Jaju

INTRODUCTION

Radiography (conventional X-ray imaging) is the recording of a shadow image of an optically opaque object using penetrating radiation and a recording medium. In 1895, Wilhelm Conrad Röntgen records the first radiography soon after he discovered one of the penetrating radiations, the X-ray (Fig. 1.1).

In conventional X-ray imaging an object is irradiated by photons generated from an X-ray source and the transmitted photons are registered on a photographic plate. Since the X-ray attenuation of the irradiated object is proportional to its electron density, the X-ray intensity transmitted after traversing a region of lower density (e.g. muscle) is greater than the X-ray intensity transmitted after traversing a region of higher density (e.g. bone). In other words, the gray level of the image recorded is inversely proportional to the attenuation of the object in the ray path. This gives contrast and thus imaging of the object as it has been applied for diagnostic purpose.[1]

This clinical method of imaging has however, some drawbacks. The three-dimensional (3D) structure of an object is collapsed onto a two-dimensional (2D) film of detector, which causes the loss of depth information. Furthermore, conventional X-ray images produce a 2D image of the anatomy only perpendicular to the X-ray beam (Fig. 1.2).

All these obstacles found its solution in the computed tomography (CT). The CT refers to the cross-sectional imaging of an object from its projection data slice by slice. The origin of the word 'tomography' is from the Greek word 'tomos' meaning 'slice' or 'section' and 'graphe' meaning 'drawing'. It is a diagnostic procedure in which a large series of cross-sectional (2D) X-ray images or tomographic slides are used to generate 3D images of the internals of an object noninvasively. Generally, the principle of CT consists of measuring the spatial distribution of a physical quantity of an object to be examined from different directions and to compute superposition free images from these data. The mathematical basis for CT was first discovered by Radon in 1917.[1]

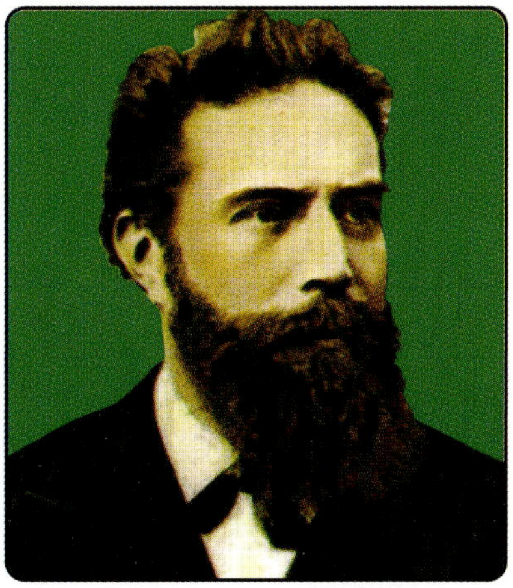

Figure 1.1: Father of radiology, Sir Wilhelm Conrad Röntgen

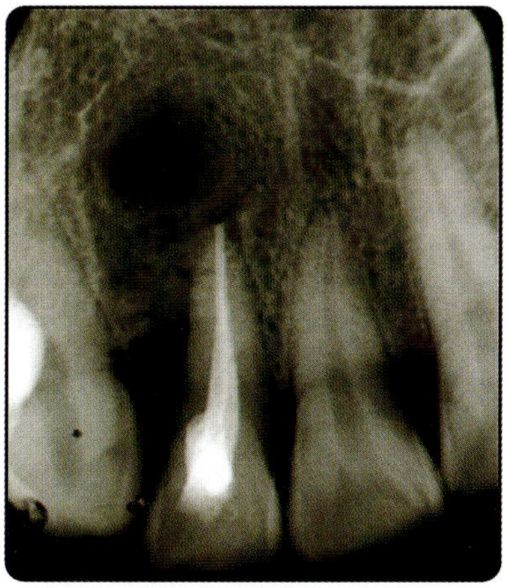

Figure 1.2: Intraoral periapical radiograph

However, it was not until 1972 that the first CT scanner was invented for which GN Hounsfield and Allan McCormack received the Nobel Prize. Since then, many improvements have been made in scanner technology as well as in the algorithms used for CT reconstruction. Cone beam computed tomography (CBCT) presents as a separate evolutionary arm to CT imaging. An early volumetric CT predecessor of CBCT, the dynamic spatial reconstructor, was developed in the late 1970s by the Biodynamics Research Unit at the Mayo Clinic. Initial interest focused primarily on applications in angiography in which soft-tissue resolution could be sacrificed in favor of high temporal and spatial resolving capabilities, CBCT prototypes based on C-arms were demonstrated as early as 1983. CBCT provided an alternate method of cross-sectional image production to fan beam CT using a comparatively less-expensive radiation detector than conventional CT. The technology transfer of CBCT to dentistry first occurred in 1995. Italian co-inventors, Attilio Tacconi and Piero Mozzo, developed a CBCT system for the maxillofacial region that was designed and produced by QR, Inc of Verona, Italy. This unit, the NewTom DVT 9000 became the first commercial CBCT unit marketed specifically to the dental market, initially introduced in Europe in 1999.[2]

DEVELOPMENT OF CBCT MACHINE

In the late 80's the diffusion of the dental implantology imposed to dentists the use of tomographic radiological examinations to program with good accuracy surgical treatments. Dental tomographs were realized to produce images of jaws cross sections by means of synchronous movement of the X-ray source and the radiographic film. Moreover, special software were created on CT machines to supply images useful to dentists (Figs 1.3 and 1.4).

Nevertheless, the poor quality of images from conventional tomographs did not allow to obtain the required information, mainly from a quantitative point of view and the CT machines were (nowadays are) predominantly dedicated to serious pathologies and were not easily available for implantology.

In those years, we held courses about radiological techniques at the University of Verona and some dentists asked us whether it would be possible to realize small CT dedicated to dentists, which were easy to use, suitable for small radiological or dental practices, and much less expensive than conventional CT.

This is how the idea of realizing a cone beam tomography was born. The capability of such a system to obtain in a unique rotation all the data necessary to reconstruct a whole volume allows to realize an unsophisticated hardware system composed by a C-arm with a low power X-ray source and a X-ray imaging detector. The C-arm rotates around the patient's head in about 60 seconds and frames are captured every degree. The X-ray detector was an image intensifier coupled with a charge-coupled device (CCD) camera. A personal computer (PC) was used to control the scan and the data acquisition and also to reconstruct the 3D volume. With the PCs available at the time of the reconstruction of a volume of 512 × 512 × 20 voxel took many hours of calculations. In the late 90's, with the arrival of 100 MHz-CPU PC, it became possible to bring to the market the first CBCT. The marketing decided to call it NewTom (Figs 1.5A and B).

The new radiological machine quickly obtained a great success, as for the first time it became easily possible for dentists to have 3D representations of the jaws, with axial and transaxial views, and also to obtain precise measurements of distances and thickness. In such a way the treatment planning became more accurate and reliable.

In the next years, the device had many important improvements, the image intensifier was replaced by a flat-panel detector and faster electronics allowed to scan the volume of interest in less than 30 seconds. Also the reconstruction time decreased until few minutes. Nowadays, CBCT is considered a standard in the field of dental radiology.

Although with little more than a decade of application in dentistry, CBCT has revolutionized oral and maxillofacial imaging.

The unit scanned the entire maxillofacial region with a volume of 15 cm × 15 cm and a complete 360° rotation for data acquisition. The detector was an image intensifier coupled with a solid-state CCD camera. At the same time, a limited volume CBCT system, scanning a cylindrical

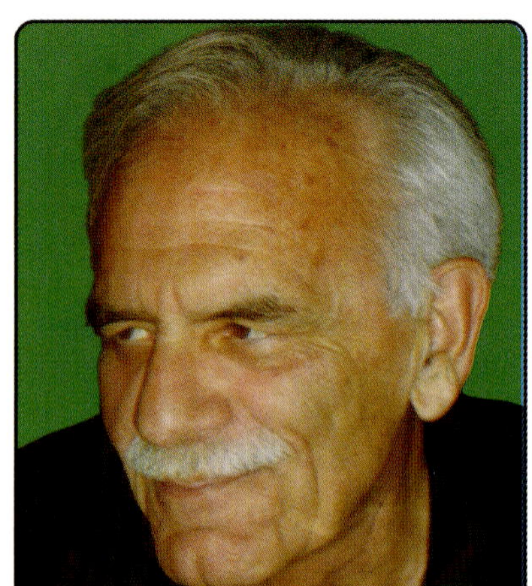

Figure 1.3: Attilio Tacconi

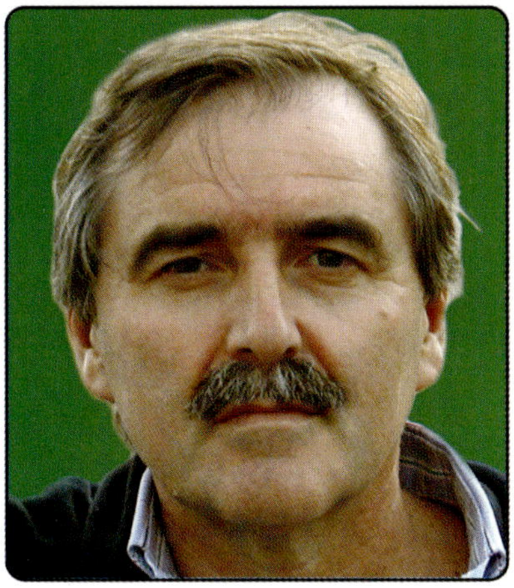

Figure 1.4: Pierluigi Mozzo

volume with a diameter of 4 cm, was under development. This prototype, called ortho-CT, was created by Arai and co-workers (1999) and based on the Scanora stand (Soredex Corporation Helsinki, Finland) with the patient in a sitting position during the examination. In 2000, actual construction of this CBCT device was transferred to J Morita MFG Corporation (Kyoto, Japan) where the 3DX limited CBCT was made ready for commercial use. In 2002, it was introduced to the European market under the name 3D Accuitomo and a year later, in March 2003, a 3D Accuitomo unit was installed at the Clinic of Oral and Maxillofacial Radiology, Public Dental Health, Göteborg, Sweden. It was equipped with an image intensifier connected to a CCD camera as detector. The X-ray field size was 3 cm × 4 cm in the rotation center and the reproduced volume thus corresponded to a cylinder of 3 cm in height and 4 cm in diameter. In August 2005, the 3D Accuitomo was replaced by a newer version, 3D Accuitomo flat-panel detector (FPD) in which a FPD is used instead of an image intensifier and a CCD camera. In this model, it is possible to choose between an X-ray field size of either 4 cm × 4 cm or 6 cm x 6 cm with reproduced volumes corresponding in size. In both versions the X-ray exposure is continuous. Commercially available CBCT systems for dentomaxillofacial imaging include the CB Mercury and CB Throne (Hitachi Medical, Kashiwa-shi, Chiba-ken, Japan), 3D Accuitomo products (J Morita manufacturing, Kyoto, Japan) and i-CAT (Xoran technologies).

Ann Arbor, Mich and Imaging Sciences International, Hatfield, PA. Similar systems designed for point-of-service head and neck imaging have also recently become available (MiniCAT, Xoran Technologies; 3D Accuitomo and 3D Accuitomo 170, J Morita Manufacturing; ILUMA cone beam CT, IMTEC, Ardmore, Okla and GE Healthcare, Chalfont Saint Giles, UK).

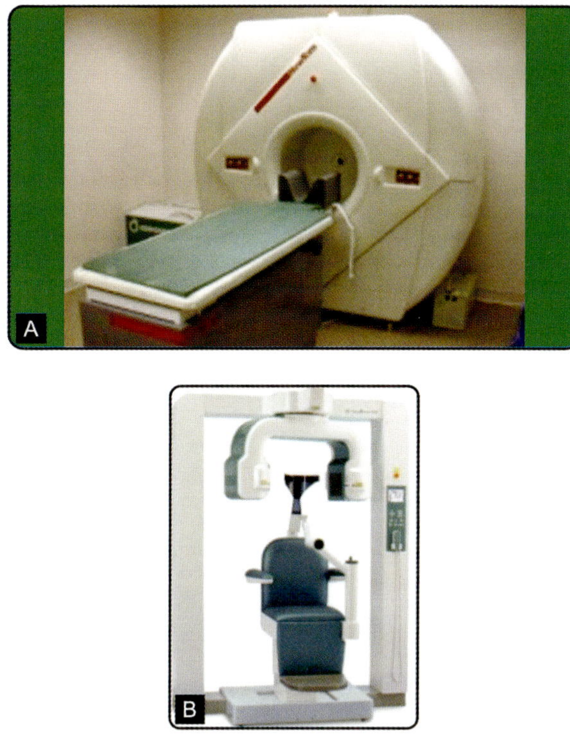

Figures 1.5A and B: NewTom DVT 9000

CONCLUSION

Dental radiology has moved a step forward with the introduction of CBCT. The CBCT imaging has given dental fraternity a diagnostic tool, which is capable of providing accurate diagnosis and treatment planning.

REFERENCES

1. Miracle AC, Mukherji SK. Conebeam CT of the head and neck, part 2: clinical applications. AJNR Am J Neuroradiol. 2009;30(7):1285-92.
2. Angelopoulos C, Scarfe WC, Farman AG. A comparison of maxillofacial CBCT and medical CT. Atlas Oral Maxillofacial Surg Clin North Am. 2012;20(1):1-17.

2

Chapter

Cone Beam Computed Tomography: Physics and Artifacts

Prashant P Jaju

INTRODUCTION

Cone beam computed tomography (CBCT) presents as a separate evolutionary arm to computed tomography (CT) imaging. An early volumetric CT predecessor of CBCT, the dynamic spatial reconstructor, was developed in the late 1970s by the Biodynamics Research Unit at the Mayo Clinic.[1] Initially CBCT was utilized for vascular imaging as early as 1983. CBCT provided an alternate method of cross-section image production to fan beam CT using a comparatively less expensive radiation detector than conventional CT.

The technology transfer of CBCT to dentistry first occurred in 1995 by two Italian co-inventors, Attilio Tacconi and Piero Mozzo. They developed a CBCT system for the maxillofacial region, which was designed and produced by QR, Inc of Verona, Italy.

This unit, the NewTom DVT 9000 became the first commercial CBCT unit marketed specifically to the dental market, initially introduced in Europe in 1999. Although with little more than a decade of application in dentistry, CBCT has revolutionized oral and maxillofacial imaging.[1]

Computed tomography is been utilized in medical and dental diagnostic field for years now. The basic principle of image acquisition and interpretation remains same with CBCT with few important improvements dedicated to dental field.

FUNDAMENTAL PRINCIPLES OF CT

The original clinical CT scanner was introduced by Sir Godfrey N Hounsfield in 1967. Data acquisition was based on a translate-rotate parallel beam geometry wherein pencil beams of X-rays were directed at a detector opposite the source and the transmitted intensity of photons incident on the detector was measured. The gantry would then both translate and rotate to capture X-ray attenuation data systematically from multiple points and angles. Image acquisition in CT has evolved through four generations of acquisition geometries. First-generation scanners used parallel pencil beams of X-rays and required both translation and rotation of the source, and a single-detector apparatus. Second-generation scanners introduced fan beam X-ray geometry and used a single-detector linear array. In third-generation scanners, the single-detector arc was introduced in conjunction with fan beam X-ray geometry. Fourth-generation scanners used a fan beam of X-rays and a circular detector array. In current practice, multidetector helical CT (MDCT) scanning is most frequently used, answering the call for reduced acquisition times. MDCT is loosely based on third-generation geometry, though the detector array has multiple rows of detectors.[2]

IMAGE ACQUISTION IN CBCT

Cone beam computed tomography imaging is performed using a rotating platform to which an X-ray source and detector are fixed. A cone-shaped source of ionizing radiation is directed through the middle of the region of interest (ROI) and the transmitted, attenuated radiation is projected onto an area X-ray detector on the opposite side. The X-ray source and detector rotate around a fulcrum, fixed within the center of the ROI. Unlike CT, the subject to be imaged does not move. This fulcrum acts as the center of the final acquired volume imaged. During the rotation, multiple sequential planar projection images covered by the detector or the field of view (FOV) are acquired in an arc of 180° or greater. These single projection transmission images constitute the raw primary data and are individually referred to as basis, frame or raw images. Basis images seem similar to cephalometric radiographic images, only each is slightly offset from the next. There are usually several hundred projection-basis images that are integrated by software to construct an image volume. The complete series of images is referred to as the projection data or volumetric dataset. Only one rotational sequence of the gantry of 180° or greater is necessary for CBCT to acquire enough data for volumetric image construction because the FOV is irradiated simultaneously.[1]

Four technological developments converged to facilitate the construction of affordable CBCT units small enough to be used in the dental office:

1. The introduction of X-ray detectors capable of rapid acquisition of multiple basis images.
2. The development of suitably resilient X-ray generators.
3. The evolution of suitable image acquisition and integration algorithms.[3,4]
4. The availability of computers powerful enough to process the enormous amount of acquired image data.

Fast data acquisition of the maxillofacial region with a single revolution, shorter examination time, and the fairly simple and inexpensive detection system are obvious advantages of CBCT that have propelled the technology for clinical applications in dentistry.

Rapid Image Acquisition in CBCT

- Improvement in X-ray detectors
- Resilient X-ray generators
- Evolution of suitable image acquisition and integration algorithms
- Powerful computers.

X-ray Generation

The X-ray generators used in CBCT machines use an operating voltage of 80–120 kVp, similar to the panoramic units. Focal spot is of the dimension 0.5–0.8 mm similar to CT machines, but with a stationary anode in CBCT. The tube current is generally much lower than CT, which reduces the power of the generator and the production of heat. Finally, in most CBCT systems, X-ray generation is pulsed to coincide with the detector activation. Pulsed X-ray beam generation is preferable because it markedly reduces total scan time and, therefore, heat production with less radiation dosage to patients. However, the low power used in this type of X-ray generator provides limitations in image quality.[1]

X-ray Detection

The detection system of both CT and CBCT scanners is responsible for recording incident X-ray photons and converting the X-ray energy to a corresponding electrical signal. This signal is represented visually as a shade of gray on the monitor display, the intensity of which should be proportional to the intensity of the incident photons at a specific point. These functions are performed by completely different detector technologies in CT and CBCT units. CBCT technology uses a X-ray detection system that is mostly dictated by the spread of the cone beam radiation. Therefore, all CBCT units use an area detector. Two systems are currently used, image intensifiers/charge-coupled device (II/CCD) and flat panel detectors (FPDs).[1]

Image Intensifiers/Charge-coupled Device

Detectors were initially produced using a configuration of image intensifiers/charge-coupled device detectors (Fig. 2.1). They consist of an X-ray image intensifier, proper optics and complementary metal oxide semiconductor (CMOS) or CCD camera. The incident X-ray beam is converted to an optical signal (light) on the input phosphor screen of the detector and to an electron beam by the photocathode inside the detector. Next the electron beam is converted to light once again (after being accelerated) at the output phosphor screen. The intensity of the light generated is adjusted by the optical iris, an integral part of the intensifier tube. Finally, the light is registered by the CMOS or CCD camera and converted to an electrical signal. The readout image includes geometric distortion and blurring generated by the image intensifier; however, correction algorithms are applied to remedy the distortion in the reconstructed image. The II/CCD detectors are large and bulky and most frequently result in circular-basis image areas (spherical volumes) rather than rectangular ones (cylindrical volumes). The main disadvantages of II/CCD detectors are geometric distortion and blurring (both inherent processes during X-ray detection).[5]

Flat Panel Detectors

Cone beam computed tomography devices now use FPD comprising an array of hydrogenated amorphous silicon thin-film transistors or, in some cases, CMOS arrays. The silicon matrix is covered by a X-ray scintillator layer, which results in an indirect X-ray detection process.[6] In both FPD circumstances, X-rays are detected indirectly by means of a scintillator such as thallium-doped cesium

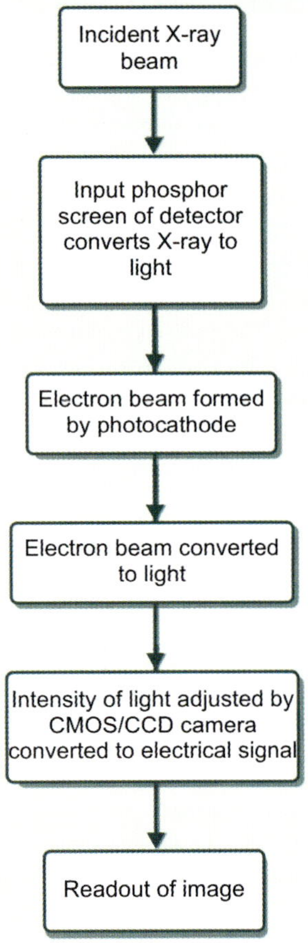

Figure 2.1: Flowchart of image intensifier/charge-coupled device (II/CCD) functioning (CMOS, complementary metal oxide semiconductor).

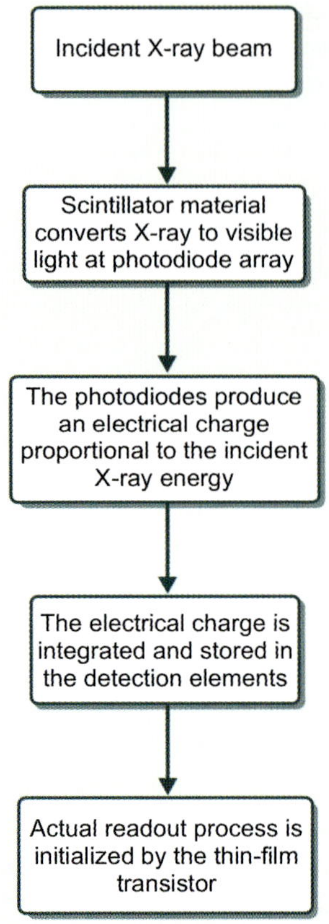

Figure 2.2: Flowchart of flat panel detector functioning

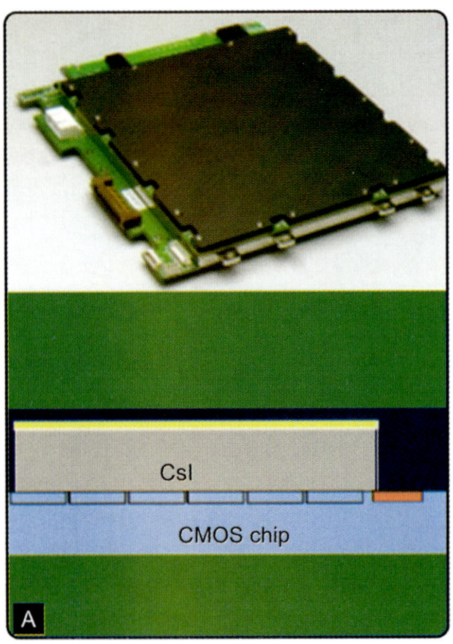

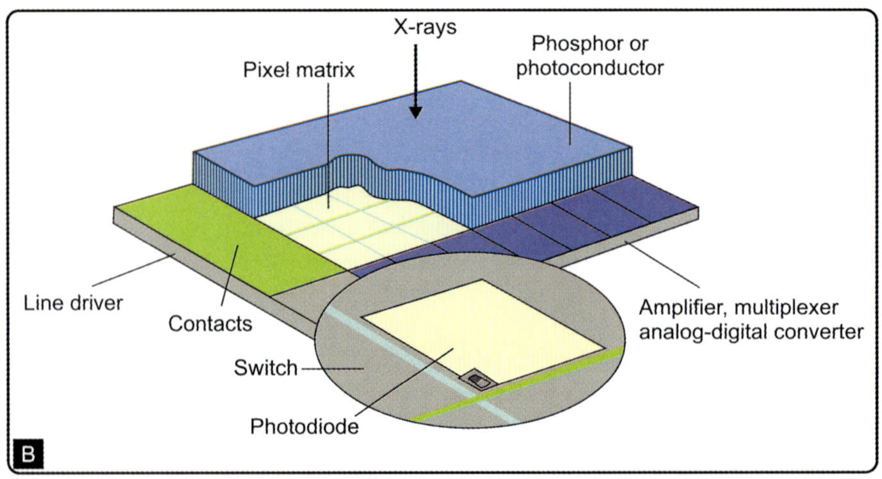

Figures 2.3A and B: Cross section of flat panel structure. *Courtesy:* Sirona Dental, Bensheim, Germany.

iodide or terbium-activated gadolinium oxysulfide, converting them to visible light that is registered in the photodiode array. The photodiodes produce an electrical charge proportional to the incident X-ray energy. The electrical charge is integrated and stored in the detection elements, which also acts as a capacitor. The actual readout process is initialized by the thin-film transistor, which switches the charge to the readout electronics via the data link (Fig. 2.2). FPDs are less complicated, less bulky and offer greater dynamic range than II/CCD detectors. FDPs also have limitations in their performance related to the linearity of response to the radiation spectrum, the uniformity of the response throughout the area of the detector and bad pixels, the effects of which on image quality are most noticeable at lower and higher exposures (Figs 2.3A and B). Baba and colleagues found FDPs to demonstrate a higher spatial resolution in comparison with the II/CCD or II/CMOS systems.[7]

Image Reconstruction

The image reconstruction stage is similar for CT and CBCT technologies. Image reconstruction in CT is a mathematical operation that converts attenuation values per voxel from X-ray projection data to grayscale images. The method used in this process has a fundamental impact on image quality and therefore, on the radiation dose to patients. There are essentially two categories of reconstruction methods, i.e. analytical reconstruction and iterative reconstruction. Operations based on filtered back projection (FBP) are one type of analytical reconstruction that is currently widely used on clinical CT scanners because of their computational efficiency and numerical stability. Different FBP-based methods have been developed for all generations of CT data-acquisition geometries including multidetector and for CBCT large-area detectors. Iterative reconstruction techniques have recently been introduced in CT imaging, because they have many advantages compared with conventional FBP techniques. Important physical factors, including focal spot and detector geometry, photon statistics, X-ray beam spectrum and scattering, can be more accurately incorporated into iterative reconstruction, yielding lower image noise and higher spatial resolution compared with FBP.[1] In addition, iterative reconstruction can reduce image artifacts such as beam hardening, windmill and metal artifacts. Iterative reconstruction may also show a significant dose reduction. However, the high computation load associated with its use has prevented its adoption in clinical CT imaging. In CBCT scanners, no control over the reconstruction method is provided to the operator.

Image Display

The volumetric data produced by CBCT is displayed soon after data acquisition and can be viewed interactively. The default presentation offered by most visualization software is usually as a series of two-dimensional (2D) contiguous interrelational images at a thickness defaulted to the native resolution in three orthogonal planes (axial, sagittal and coronal). Regarding MDCT display, data are usually transferred from the acquisition workstation to a separate console, where it is formatted. However, in CBCT, imaging acquisition and visualization are usually performed on the same computer. Display software provides an almost infinite and perhaps bewildering number of visualization options, each directed toward highlighting specific components of the volumetric data set.[1]

Multiplanar Reformation[8]

Because of the isotropic nature of the volumetric data sets, they can be sectioned nonorthogonally. Most software provides for various non-axial 2D images, referred to as multiplanar reformation (MPR). Such MPR modes include oblique, curved planar reformation (providing 'simulated' distortion-free panoramic images) and serial transplanar reformation (providing cross sections), all of which can be used to highlight specific anatomic regions and diagnostic tasks, which is important, given the complex structure of the maxillofacial region. Because of the large number of component orthogonal images in each plane and the difficulty in relating adjacent structures, two methods have been developed to visualize adjacent voxels.

Ray Sum or Ray Casting

Any multiplanar image can be 'thickened' by increasing the number of adjacent voxels included in the display, which creates an image slab that represents a specific volume of the patient, referred to as a ray sum. Full-thickness perpendicular ray sum images can be used to generate simulated projections such as lateral cephalometric images. Unlike conventional X-rays, these ray sum images are without magnification and are undistorted. However, this technique uses the entire volumetric data set and interpretation suffers from the problems of 'anatomic noise,' the superimposition of multiple structures.[8]

Three-dimensional Volume Rendering

Volume rendering refers to techniques that allow the visualization of three-dimensional (3D) data through integration of large volumes of adjacent voxels and selective display. Two specific techniques are available.

Indirect volume rendering: It is a complex process; requiring selecting the intensity or density of the grayscale level of the voxels to be displayed within an entire data set (called segmentation). This technique is technically demanding and computationally difficult, requiring specific software; however, it provides a volumetric surface reconstruction with depth.

Direct volume rendering: Clinically and technically, direct volume rendering is a much more simple process. The most common direct volume rendering technique is maximum intensity projection (MIP). MIP visualizations are achieved by evaluating each voxel value along an imaginary projection ray from the observer's eyes within a particular volume of interest and then representing only the highest value as the display value. Voxel intensities that are below an arbitrary threshold are eliminated.[8]

FIELD OF VIEW

Field of view could be defined as area of interest to be covered during the scanning procedure. One major advantage of most CBCT units in comparison with CT is the ability to reduce the FOV to the ROI, either mechanically or electronically. Mechanical reduction in the dimensions of the X-ray beam can be achieved by either preirradiation (reducing primary radiation dimensions) or postirradiation (reducing the dimensions of the transmitted radiation before it is detected) collimation. Currently most units use adjustable lead shields as primary collimation at the radiation source. Electronic collimation involves the elimination of data recorded on the detector that is peripheral to the area of interest. In this case, there is no physical reduction in irradiation of the ROI by physical means; the full FOV is exposed, but only the selected region is recorded. Both techniques reduce the amount of data for computational purposes and reduce reconstruction time; however, only preirradiation physical collimation of the X-ray beam limits X-ray radiation exposure to the ROI and results in reduced patient irradiation.[8]

The dimensions of the FOV depend primarily on the detector size and shape, the beam projection geometry and the ability to collimate the beam. Field size limitation therefore ensures that an optimal FOV can be selected for each patient, based on disease presentation and the region designated to be imaged.

The CBCT systems can be categorized according to the available FOV or selected scan volume height as follows:

1. Localized region: Approximately 5 cm or less (e.g. dentoalveolar, temporomandibular joint).
2. Single arch: 5–7 cm (e.g. maxilla or mandible).
3. Interarch: 7–10 cm (e.g. mandible and superiorly to include the inferior concha).
4. Maxillofacial: 10–15 cm (e.g. mandible and extending to nasion).
5. Craniofacial: Greater than 15 cm (e.g. from the lower border of the mandible to the vertex of the head).

Extended FOV scanning incorporating the craniofacial region is difficult to incorporate into cone beam design, because of the high cost of large-area detectors. The expansion of scan volume height has been accomplished by one unit (i-CAT extended FOV model) by the software addition of two rotational scans to produce a single volume with 22 cm height.[8]

Depending upon the FOV radiation dose are as follows:

- Large FOV: 68–1073 μSv (Table 2.1)
- Medium FOV: 69–560 μSv (Table 2.2)
- Small FOV: 189–652 μSv (Table 2.3).

Selection of appropriate FOV according to application thus has to be selected.

Table 2.1: Large field of view (FOV) machines (> 15 cm)

Model	Manufacturer	Maximum FOV (cm)	Minimum voxel (mm)
i-CAT FLX	Imaging Sciences International	17 × 23	0.125
Classic i-CAT	Imaging Sciences International	16 × 22	0.2
NewTom 3G	QR Srl	20 × 20	0.2
CB MercuRay	Hitachi Medical	20 × 20	0.2
Kodak 9500	CareStream	18 × 21	0.2
ProMax 3D max	Planmeca	16 × 23	0.1
Master 3DS	Vatech	19 × 20	0.164

IMAGE QUALITY

Image quality has two elements, subjective and objective. In dentistry, subjective image quality is usually obtained from averaging observer ratings of clarity in visibility of specific anatomic structures (e.g. periodontal ligament space or trabecular pattern in the mandible). Objective assessment of image quality, at least in CT, is based on quantitative measurements of particular patterns in a test object. These measurements include CT number correlation, contrast resolution, image homogeneity and uniformity, point spread or modulation transfer function and metal

Table 2.2: Medium field of view (FOV) machines (8–15 cm)

Model	Manufacturer	Maximum FOV (cm)	Minimum voxel (mm)
Galileos	Sirona	15 × 15	0.15
NewTom VGi	QR Srl	15 × 15	0.075
CS 9300	CareStream	13.5 × 17	0.09
ProMax 3D Mid	Planmeca	9 × 16	0.1
i-CAT	Imaging Sciences International	8 × 14	0.125
SkyView	MyRay	15 × 15	0.16
Scanora 3D	Soredex	7.5 × 14.5	0.133
Picasso Trio	Vatech	7 × 12	0.2

Table 2.3: Small field of view (FOV) machines (< 8 cm)

Model	Manufacturer	Maximum FOV (cm)	Minimum voxel (mm)
Orthophos XG 3D	Sirona	8 × 8/5 × 5	0.1
3D Accuitomo	J Morita	3 × 4/6 × 6/8 × 8	0.125
Kodak 9000 3D	CareStream	4 × 5	0.076
ProMax 3D	Planmeca	8 × 8	0.1
GXDP-700	Gendex	6 × 8	0.2
CB Throne	Hitachi Medical	10 × 10	0.125
Cranex 3D	Soredex	6 × 8	0.2
PaX-Uni3D	Vatech	5 × 8	0.08

artifacts; however, no such tool has been accepted for image quality assessment in CBCT. Because of these differences, few investigators have directly compared image quality of comparable objects using both CBCT and CT.[9]

Image Resolution

There are two types of image resolution; spatial resolution, determining the proximity of details able to be recorded separately, and contrast resolution, enabling distinction between tissues of different radiodensity.

Spatial Resolution

Spatial resolution is the ability of the imaging system to distinguish small structures that lie close to one another. It is an important parameter, because it is directly linked to diagnostic efficiency. Spatial resolution in CT imaging is ultimately dependent on the shape and size of the voxels that compose the imaging volume. CBCT units, in general, provide voxel resolutions that are isotropic (equal in all 3 orthogonal dimensions). The spatial resolution of CBCT systems is primarily a function of the nominal pixel size on the area detector's factors such as beam projection geometry, patient scatter, detector motion blur and fill factor, focal spot size, number of basis images and reconstruction algorithm, all contribute to the final maximum achievable resolution. The resolution of the area detector is submillimeter (range 0.07–0.4 mm), which results in submillimeter voxel size.[8]

As a result, the spatial resolution of CBCT images is identical in all three planes. The inherent isotropy of the CBCT volume voxels facilitates accurate multiplanar reconstructions of similar resolution to the acquired resolution and smooth volumetric reconstructions. This accuracy seems to place CBCT in an advantageous position in comparison with CT, whereby isotropy or near isotropy is determined by proper section thickness selection. CBCT generally demonstrates a high spatial resolution with a low radiation dose. The reported resolution of contemporary CBCT scanners is almost 5 line pairs per millimeter (lp/mm), whereas the spatial resolution of CT scanners is lower and approximately 2–3 lp/mm.

Contrast Resolution

Contrast resolution is the ability of an imaging system to distinguish minor differences in tissue attenuation and to display them with different gray levels. It is measured in Hounsfield units (HU), which is the relative density of body tissues according to a calibrated grayscale level, based on normalized, HU values for air (–1,000 HU), water (0 HU) and dense bone (+1,000 HU). CBCT systems have been reported to demonstrate contrast discernment typically in the range of 10 HU. When compared with CBCT, CT systems demonstrate superior contrast detectability, which approaches 1 HU. The limited contrast resolution of CBCT technology makes it difficult to depict different soft tissue structures (e.g. muscle and glands or blood vessels) as in images of the floor of the mouth or the maxillofacial region, which are of great interest to the oral and maxillofacial surgeon; this renders current CBCT machines unsuitable for diagnosis, when soft tissue contrast is of great importance.[1]

Several factors limit the contrast resolution of CBCT. The inherent geometric configuration of image acquisition involving an area detector to register attenuated primary radiation from a cone source produces significant scatter radiation. This scatter radiation contributes to the increased noise of the image as well as being a significant factor in reducing the contrast of any CBCT system. In addition, because of the divergence of the X-ray beam over the area detector, there is a large variation or nonuniformity of the incident X-ray beam on patients. Subsequently, there is resultant nonuniformity in absorption on the area detector, with greater signal-to-noise (SNR) intensity on the cathode side of the image relative to the anode side (heel effect). Further, the dynamic range of area detectors in both FPD and II/CCD configurations used in CBCT imaging is generally inferior to that of CT detectors.[10] For these reasons, and the reduced operating kilovolt (peak) and milliampere of CBCT compared with CT, maxillofacial CBCT images lack adequate grayscale sensitivity to discern subtle differences between soft tissues such as between fluids and solid tumors.

Image Noise

Image noise refers to the density differences in a radiographic image that are attributed to statistical fluctuations on the distribution of the X-ray photons registered by the detector. Noise is of great importance as a determinant of the quality of an image. Uneven distribution of X-ray photons may alter the appearance of a region in the imaging volume by producing inhomogeneity of the gray levels and may affect diagnostic efficiency. The SNR is a measure of noise and refers to the amount of radiation reaching the detector (signal) over noise (statistical fluctuations). Voxel size and radiation exposure are the main factors affecting noise. When smaller voxel sizes are selected, the fluctuation in the distribution of the X-ray photons on the detector is increased and fewer X-rays (signal) reach the detector elements. Consequently, noise is increased and the SNR is low. Current CBCT scanners can acquire data at voxel sizes that range from 0.08 mm to 0.4 mm, which results in high levels of noise, given the fact that the radiation dose with CBCT systems is generally low. Although requirements exist for sharp and high-detail images, smaller voxel sizes should be selected only based on the diagnostic task at hand, because they will suffer great levels of noise. SNR is considerably higher with CT systems. This factor is mainly because the slice thickness in these systems is rarely less than 0.5 mm and because of the higher radiation dose. Higher-resolution images unavoidably require higher radiation exposures to reduce the proportion of inhomogeneity in the X-ray beam and reduce image noise.

ARTIFACTS IN CBCT

In CT, the term artifact is applied to any systematic discrepancy between the CT numbers in the reconstructed image and the true attenuation coefficients of the object. CT images are inherently more prone to artifacts than conventional radiographs, because the image is reconstructed from something on the order of a million independent detector measurements. The presence of gray level nonuniformities in CBCT contributes to artifact formation in reconstructed CBCT images. These artifacts contribute to image degradation and can lead to inaccurate or false diagnoses. Some of these artifacts are more pronounced in CBCT units than their CT counterparts, because of the different processes in which the images are acquired (Fig. 2.4).

Artifact relating to CBCT is divided into three main categories, physics based, patient based and scanner based. Physics-based artifacts result from the physical processes involved in the acquisition of CT data. Patient-based artifacts are caused by factors related to the patient's form or function. Scanner-based artifacts result from imperfections in scanner function.

Physics-based Artifacts

Noise

Noise is defined as an unwanted, randomly and/or nonrandomly distributed disturbance of a signal that tends to obscure the signal's information content from the observer. Noise affects images produced by CBCT units by reducing low contrast resolution, making it difficult to differentiate low-density tissues thereby reducing the ability to segment effectively. The noise in traditional projection radiography is primarily from quantum mottle, which is defined as a variation in image density due to statistical fluctuation of photon fluency in the radiation field. In well-designed X-ray systems, the quantum noise is governed by the number of X-ray photons absorbed in the detector, the higher the number of photons absorbed, the lower the quantum mottle. The number of X-ray photons emitted is directly related to

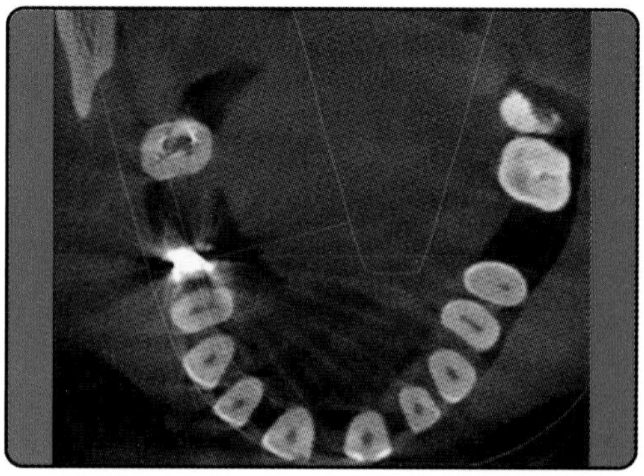

Figure 2.4: Image degradation of axial cone beam computed tomography (CBCT) slice due to metallic restoration

the mA of the X-ray unit. Another source of noise in CT is scattered radiation. Scattered radiation arises from interactions of the primary radiation beam with the atoms in the object being imaged and its magnitude is largely dependent on patient size, shape and position in the scan field. It is a major source of image degradation in X-ray imaging techniques. Quantum noise is fundamentally related to image quality and is a function of dose, tissue transmissivity and voxel size. Noise is, in turn, a principal determinant of contrast resolution and, to a lesser extent, spatial resolution, which, along with artifacts, constitute the major observable determinants of overall image quality (Fig. 2.5).

The CBCT imaging with FPD technology typically affords excellent spatial resolution with a relatively low patient dose. Contrast resolution suffers, however, due to increased X-ray scatter and the reduced temporal resolution and dynamic range of the FPDs. Increased scatter not only amplifies patient dose but also is a principal contributor to reduced contrast resolution and increased noise in CBCT images.[11]

Beam Hardening

An X-ray beam is composed of individual photons with a range of energies. As the beam passes through an object, it becomes 'harder', that is to say its mean energy increases, because the lower energy photons are absorbed more rapidly than the higher energy photons. Two types of artifact can result from this effect, so-called cupping artifacts and the appearance of dark bands or streaks between dense objects in the image.

Cupping artifacts from beam hardening occur, when X-rays passing through the center of a large object become harder than those passing through the edges of the object due to the greater amount of material the beam has to penetrate. Because the beam becomes harder in the center of the object, the resultant profile of the linear attenuation coefficients appears as a 'cup'. The cupping effect artifact is demonstrated, when a uniform cylindrical object is imaged. As the effects of beam hardening and scatter are most prevalent in the center of a cylindrical object, it is this area that is dominated by the cupping effect artifact.

The second type of artifact relating to beam hardening is dark streaks and bands between dense objects in an image. In dental imaging, this type of artifact can be seen between two implants located in the same jaw that are in close proximity to each other (Fig. 2.6).

This occurs because the portion of the beam that passes through both objects at certain tube positions becomes harder than when it passes through only one of the objects at other tube positions. It is well known that an artifact referred to as the 'truncation artifact' or 'truncated-view artifact' is inherent to CBCT imaging. This artifact occurs because the size of the FOV used in CBCT is smaller than the size of the object being imaged. The largest error due to the truncated-view artifact will occur near the edge of the FOV. Manufacturers minimize beam hardening by using filtration, antiscatter grids, calibration correction and beam hardening correction software.[11]

Filtration: The use of filtration to decrease beam hardening can be achieved by utilizing filtering materials like aluminum, copper, tin or Thoraeus filters. The bow tie or wedge filter is the prototypical compensating filter used in CBCT systems. It modulates the beam profile by increasing photon density at the center of the cone and decrementally reducing density at the periphery. Compensating filtration is not without criticism, however, because beam hardness has been shown to negatively impact detector efficiency, as demonstrated by a decrease in the ratio of the output SNR to the entrance exposure (SNR/entrance exposure).[11]

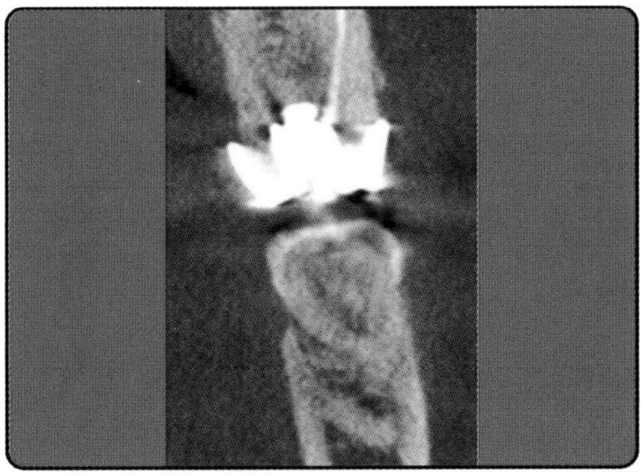

Figure 2.5: Noise reducing image contrast

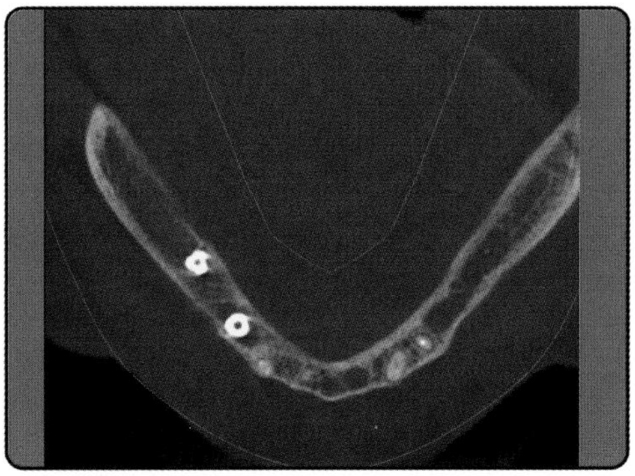

Figure 2.6: Dark streaks and bands between two implants

Antiscatter grids: It represents an alternative method of direct scatter reduction that has been used with FPDs in digital radiographic and fluoroscopic imaging for some time. Rather than modulating the beam properties at the source, a grid of lead leaves is fitted over the detector to preferentially absorb off-axis radiation not contributing to primary photon fluence.

In CBCT systems, the lead leaves are arranged in a radial pattern centered on the focal spot of the FPD. Antiscatter grids have been evaluated in several experimental CBCT systems with mixed results. A reduction in both cupping artifact and overall scatter has been observed, though there may be insufficient improvement in contrast and observed image quality to warrant use except in situations of high scatter. For a relatively small FOVs such as that used in a targeted head and neck scan, antiscatter grids may improve image contrast and reduce cupping artifacts, but the increased noise requires that the dose be increased or spatial resolution be decreased to produce a high-quality image.[11]

Calibration: Manufacturers calibrate their scanners using phantoms in a range of sizes. This allows the detectors to be calibrated with compensation tailored for the beam hardening effects of different parts of the patient.

Software corrections: Beam hardening correction software is an iterative correction algorithm may be applied, when images of bony regions are being reconstructed. This helps to minimize blurring of the bone-soft tissue interface in brain scans and also reduces the appearance of dark bands in non-homogeneous cross sections.[11]

Patient-based Artifacts

Metal Artifacts

The presence of metal objects in the scan field can lead to severe streaking artifacts. They occur because the density of the metal is beyond the normal range that can be handled by the computer, resulting in incomplete attenuation profiles. Metallic objects such as dental restorations, surgical plates, dental implants and pins, and radiographic markers can cause this type of the artifact. Since the metal in these materials highly attenuate the X-ray beam, the attenuation values of objects behind the object are incorrectly high. Due to the reconstruction of the cone beam image, the metal causes the effect of bright and dark streaks in CT images, which significantly degrade the image quality. In conventional CT images metallic artifacts traverse the object in the direction of the gantry and only at the level of the high attenuation object. In CBCT, the metallic streak artifacts occur in all directions from the high attenuation object because of the cone-shaped beam (Fig. 2.7).[11]

Software corrections for metal artifacts

Streaking caused by over ranging can be greatly reduced by means of special software corrections. Manufacturers use a variety of interpolation techniques to substitute the over range values in attenuation profiles. Metal artifact reduction software (MARS) provided by Sirona (Germany), is one such metal reduction software, which improves the quality of image. The usefulness of metal artifact reduction software is sometimes limited because, although streaking distant from the metal implants is removed, there still remains a loss of detail around the metal-tissue interface, which is often the main area of diagnostic interest. Beam hardening correction software should also be used, when scanning metal objects to minimize the additional artifacts due to beam hardening.

Motion Artifacts

Patient motion can cause misregistration artifacts within the image. Because of the relatively long acquisition times (compared to conventional radiography) and volumetric image acquisition, motion artifacts are common in CBCT. These artifacts can be attributed to improper patient stabilization. Small motions cause image blurring and larger physical displacements. They produce artifacts that appear as double images or ghost images. This results in poor overall image quality. Since the resolutions of the present CBCT are very high, ranging from 0.08 mm to 0.4 mm, even small motions can have a detrimental effect on image quality. The use of positioning aids is sufficient to prevent voluntary movement in most patients.[11]

Scanner-based Artifacts

Ring Artifacts

If one of the detectors is out of calibration on a scanner, the detector will give a consistently erroneous reading at each

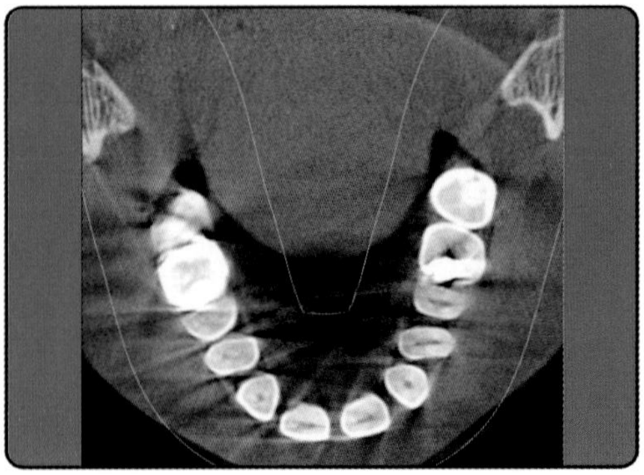

Figure 2.7: Artifacts due to metallic restorations

Table 2.4: Equivalent dose to tissues/organs (in Sv) in the head and neck from CBCT* and MDCT† examinations

Values from RANDO phantom	Bone marrow	Thyroid	Esophagus	Skin	Bone surface	Salivary glands	Brain[1,2]	Lymphatic nodes[1]	Extrathoracic region[1]	Muscle[1,2]	Oral mucosa[1]
NewTom 3G large FOV‡ [3]	125	333	57	62	581	956	700	42	826	42	915
CB MercuRay maximum quality[3]	1,542	10,042	622	788	7,153	11,833	9,275	536	10,633	536	11,226
CB MercuRay P FOV standard quality[3]	692	6,333	393	389	3,211	5,467	3,967	256	5,036	256	5,211
Next Generation i-CAT portrait mode[4]	147	183	33	52	294	1,250	950	54	1,083	54	1,226
CB MercuRay P FOV[3]	940	1,700	177	641	4,360	10,561	5,933	430	8,736	430	10,111
Classic i-CAT standard FOV	95	267	30	54	149	1,450	567	61	1,224	61	1,422
Next Generation i-CAT landscape mode[4]	105	283	45	82	211	1,836	808	76	1,537	76	1,776
Iluma standard	161	350	50	82	745	1,661	1,267	72	1,455	72	1,630
Iluma ultra	834	1,733	233	421	3,869	8,400	6,267	363	7,433	363	8,289
Galileos default exposure	82	233	37	40	382	1,606	267	68	1,283	68	1,556
Galileos maximum exposure	150	450	47	77	696	2,900	467	125	2,362	125	2,896
Somatom 64 MDCT	1,031	3,700	1,560	619	4,785	15,300	7,100	696	13,514	696	14,878
Somatom 64 MDCT w/Care Dose 4D	697	2,350	740	501	3,151	8,667	5,750	408	8,357	408	8,789
CB MercuRay I FOV maxillary arch[3]	466	1,300	110	344	2,161	9,006	2,950	383	7,769	383	9,078
ProMax 3D small adult	468	1,267	120	339	2,170	12,939	600	543	9,631	543	13,285
ProMax 3D large adult	592	1,783	207	382	2,747	17,539	800	719	12,731	719	17,581
PreXion 3D standard	164	683	53	135	760	4,761	383	192	3,805	192	4,704
PreXion 3D high resolution estimates based on $CTDI_{vol}$ data	325	1,800	133	264	1,508	9,372	783	375	7,183	375	9,085
Somatom 64 MDCT	597	0	1,270	635	2,770	12,700	0	635	12,700	635	12,700
Somatom 64 MDCT w/Care Dose 4D	383	0	728	520	1,776	7,700	0	389	8,352	389	7,793

*CBCT, cone beam computed tomography; †MDCT, multidetector helical computed tomography; ‡FOV, field of view. ***Reprint with permission*** from Ludlow JB, Ivanovice M.[15]

Note: 1, International Commission on Radiological Protection (ICRP) 2007; 2, ICRP 1990; 3, Previously published data; 4, average of 2 dosimeter runs.

angular position, resulting in a circular artifact. A scanner with solid-state detectors, where all the detectors are separate entities, is in principle more susceptible to ring artifacts. Rings visible in a uniform phantom or in air might not be visible on a clinical image, if a wide window is used. Even if they are visible, they would rarely be confused with disease. However, they can impair the diagnostic quality of an image and this is particularly likely when central detectors are affected, creating a dark smudge at the center of the image. Currently there is no evidence of ring artifacts on CBCT machine in dental radiology literature.[11]

RADIATION DOSE

Dose-reduction techniques should always be addressed in association with diagnostic quality. Generally in CT, the higher the exposure parameters (mA, kVp), the greater the number of sections (thinner slices) and the larger the FOV, the higher the radiation exposure to patients. Similarly for CBCT, exposure parameters and FOV determine patient dose. However, in addition, continuous exposure units and higher numbers of basis images also increase exposure. Therefore, it is imperative for operators of both technologies to use specific exposure imaging protocols that provide images with sufficient image quality to answer a specific diagnostic concern with the least amount of radiation. This concept is called as low as reasonably achievable (ALARA) and is equally applicable to both technologies. In dentistry, the specialty of oral and maxillofacial radiology [(American Academy of Oral and Maxillofacial Radiology (AAOMR), www.aaomr.org] has published position statements on the appropriate use of CBCT,[12] and recently, a specific document addressing CBCT in endodontics. Ludlow and Ivanovic reported that, in general, effective doses for CBCT devices decreased with smaller FOV scans. Smaller FOV helps in achieving a substantial dose reduction. It has been demonstrated that reducing the height of the FOV by a third nearly halves the radiation dose. Smaller FOV also reduces the scatter radiation. A small FOV is preferred in the assessment of a single implant site, a third molar, supernumerary teeth and localized lesions.[13]

Large FOV CBCT E2007 ranged from 68 to 1,073 μSv and medium FOV E2007 ranged from 69 to 560 μSv. At a comparable medium FOV, a 64-slice MDCT (Somatom Sensation, Siemens Medical Solutions USA, Malvern, Pennsylvania) produced 530 μSv at default settings and 860 μSv using a dose-sparing protocol (automatic exposure control). A large FOV is commonly used in orthodontic treatment planning, orthognathic surgical planning, fitting of bridges or dentures and cases of trauma.[13]

Loubele and colleagues reported very low E2007 for 3 CBCT scanners (range, 13–82 μSv) and appreciably higher doses for 2 MDCT scanners (range 474–1,160 μSv) they examined.[14] More recently, these studies demonstrate that CBCT technologies seem to provide reduced doses as compared with CT. Despite the lower doses of CBCT, strict adherence to selection criteria, imaging protocols and ALARA is strongly recommended. Using these technologies as a screening diagnostic tool in dentistry is fundamentally incorrect (Table 2.4).

CONCLUSION

To understand any imaging modalities, it is of paramount importance to know about the principle, functioning, role of each components and its influence on the image quality. This chapter has highlighted all these parameters in great details, thus clearing the ground for understanding the applications of CBCT in subsequent chapters.

REFERENCES

1. Angelopoulos C, Scarfe WC, Farman AG. A comparison of maxillofacial CBCT and medical CT. Atlas Oral Maxillofac Surg Clin North Am. 2012;20(1):1-17.
2. Miracle AC, Mukherji SK. Conebeam CT of the head and neck, part 1: physical principles. AJNR Am J Neuroradiol. 2009;30(6):1088-95.
3. Feldkamp LA, Davis LC, Kress JW. Practical cone-beam algorithm. J Opt Soc Am A. 1984;1:612–9.
4. Wischmann HA, Luijendijk HA, Meulenbrugge HJ, et al. Correction of amplifier nonlinearity, offset, gain, temporal artifacts and defects for flat-panel digital imaging devices. In: Antonuk LE, Yaffe MJ (Eds). Medical Imaging 2002: Physics of Medical Imaging—proceedings of SPIE, vol. 4682. San Diego (CA): SPIE; 2002. pp. 427-37.
5. Baba R, Ueda K, Okabe M. Using a flat-panel detector in high resolution cone beam CT for dental imaging. Dentomaxillofac Radiol. 2004;33(5):285-90.
6. Jaffray DA, Siewerdsen JH. Cone-beam computed tomography with a flat panel imager: initial performance characterization. Med Phys. 2000;27(6):1311-23.
7. Baba R, Konno Y, Ueda K, et al. Comparison of flat-panel detector and image intensifier detector for cone-beam CT. Comput Med Imaging Graph. 2002;26(3):153-8.
8. Scarfe WC, Farman AG. What is cone-beam CT and how does it work? Dent Clin North Am. 2008;52(4):707-30.
9. Suomalainen A, Kiljunen T, Käser Y, et al. Dosimetry and image quality of four dental cone beam computed tomography scanners compared with multislice computed tomography scanners. Dentomaxillofac Radiol. 2009;38(6):367-78.
10. Gupta R, Grasruck M, Suess C, et al. Ultra-high resolution flat-panel volume CT: fundamental principles, design

architecture and system characterization. Eur Radiol. 2006;16(6):1191-205.

11. Jaju P, Jain M, Singh A, et al. Artifacts in cone beam CT. OJST. 2013;3:292-7.
12. Carter L, Farman AG, Geist J, et al. American Academy of Oral and Maxillofacial Radiology executive opinion statement on performing and interpreting diagnostic cone beam computed tomography. Oral Surg Oral Med Oral Pathol Oral Radiol Endod. 2008;106(4):561-2.
13. Chau AC, Fung K. Comparison of radiation dose for implant imaging using conventional spiral tomography, computed tomography, and cone-beam computed tomography. Oral Surg Oral Med Oral Pathol Oral Radiol Endod. 2009;107(4):559-65.
14. Loubele M, Bogaerts R, Van Dijck E, et al. Comparison between effective radiation dose of CBCT and MSCT scanners for dentomaxillofacial applications. Eur J Radiol. 2009;71(3):461-8.
15. Ludlow JB, Ivanovic M. Comparative dosimetry of dental CBCT devices and 64-slice CT for oral and maxillofacial radiology. Oral Surg Oral Med Oral Pathol Oral Radiol Endod. 2008;106(1):106-14.

3 Chapter

Need of Cone Beam Computed Tomography in Dentistry

Prashant V Suvarna

LIMITATION OF TWO-DIMENSIONAL IMAGING

Diagnostic imaging modality in all aspects of dentistry begins with the basic, easily available two-dimensional (2D) conventional technique like intraoral radiography including occlusal radiography and orthopantomography. Although, intraoral periapical radiography are inexpensive, readily available and provide highest resolution images, they are unable to unveil the third dimension, i.e. buccolingual dimension and undercuts due to superimposition because of their inherent projection technique. Early changes in pathology cannot be appreciated due to superimposition of cortical plates. It also exhibits distortion at various anatomic areas leading to improper vertical height estimation. Occlusal radiography to assess the buccolingual dimension too fails as peripheral edges of the bone visible, represent the contour of the widest portion of the bone, which is at the base rather than the apical portion of the alveolar ridge. Orthopantomography has the inherent limitation of being 2D with inherent horizontal and vertical distortion.

Two-dimensional imaging has served dentistry well and will continue to do so for the foreseeable future, taking into account its easy availability and cost efficiency. However, the emerging technology and its advancement in application will eradicate the disadvantages of conventional technique to dispel the darkness of imagination, and illuminate to visualize the real life-like images.

Then, entering into the era of three-dimensional (3D) imaging computed tomography (CT) scan came to rescue and provided us with the third dimension, but the situation was operated by general radiologists with no particular interest or training in dental radiology, or pathology. Because there was less interaction between the various specialties of dentistry and the radiologist, the optimal use was not accomplished. Dental radiologists who were experts in anatomy of jaws and sensitive to the needs of the dental specialists did not have access to the CT scanners.

THREE-DIMENSIONAL IMAGING

Imagine a technology that can be easily used by a dental radiologist, which brings the most detailed knowledge of the patient's dental anatomy and greater treatment predictability right into the dental office. A good imagination is no longer necessary to achieve this goal. The technology, cone beam computed tomography (CBCT) imaging, is not just a dental daydream but also an everyday reality in many dental offices nationally and internationally. 3D technology is already redefining dental outcomes across a broad spectrum of treatment options including implants, bone grafting, oral surgery, orthodontics and endodontics. The ability to capture a 3D image of the mouth and to view it from all angles together with the capability of rotating the 3D mode and zooming in on details can only result in more effective dental treatment.

The recent introduction of CBCT to dentistry represents a true shift from a 2D 'planar' approach of dental radiography to a 3D 'volumetric' approach. These systems, specifically designed for the maxillofacial region, provide comprehensive, accurate and undistorted images of the hard tissues of the jaws, teeth and related anatomical structures. The CBCT has increased accuracy, higher resolution, reduced scan time, a reduction in radiation dose and reduced cost for the patient. With submillimeter accuracy, CBCT has created much excitement by expanding the role of imaging from pure diagnosis to image-guided treatments and custom appliance fabrication. The CBCT easily surpasses the shortcomings of 2D as well as 3D imaging techniques like CT.

X-RAY BEAM LIMITATION

Reducing the size of the irradiated area by collimation of the primary X-ray beam to the area of interest minimizes the radiation dose. Due to multiple field of view (FOV) options now available in CBCT machines, small-to-entire craniofacial regions can be scanned depending upon the indication. This significantly reduces the X-ray beam size.[1]

IMAGE ACCURACY

The volumetric data set comprises a 3D block of smaller cuboid structures known as voxels, each representing a specific degree of X-ray absorption. The size of these voxels determines the resolution of the image. In conventional CT, the voxels are anisotropic rectangular cubes, where the longest dimension of the voxel is the axial slice thickness and is determined by slice pitch, a function of gantry motion. Although, CT voxel surfaces can be as small as 0.625 mm^2, their depth is usually in the order of 1–2 mm. All CBCT units provide voxel resolutions that are isotropic—equal in all three orientations. This produces submillimeter resolution (often exceeding the highest grade multislice CT) ranging from 0.4 mm to as low as 0.125 mm.[1] Hence, dental applications such as endodontics have received tremendous boost in diagnosis and subsequent treatment planning.

RAPID SCAN TIME

Because CBCT acquires all basic images in a single rotation, scan time is rapid (10–70 s) and comparable with that of medical spiral multidetector computed tomography (MDCT). Although faster scanning time usually means fewer basic images from which to reconstruct the volumetric data set, motion artifacts due to subject movement are reduced and also reduction in the radiation dose delivered to the patient.[1]

DOSE REDUCTION

Published reports indicate that the effective dose of radiation [average range 36.9–50.3 microsievert (μSv)] is significantly reduced by up to 98% compared with CT systems (average range for mandible 1,320–3,324 μSv; average range for maxilla 1,031–1,420 μSv). This reduces the effective patient dose to approximately that of a film-based periapical survey of the dentition (13–100 μSv) or 4–15 times that of a single panoramic radiograph (2.9–11 μSv).[2-6]

DISPLAY MODES UNIQUE TO MAXILLOFACIAL IMAGING

Access and interaction with medical CT data are not possible, as workstations are required. Although such data can be 'converted' and imported into proprietary programs for use on personal computers (e.g. SimPlant, Materialise, Leuven, Belgium), this process is expensive and requires an intermediary stage that can extend the diagnostic phase. Reconstruction of CBCT data is performed natively by a personal computer. In addition, software can be made available to the user, not just the radiologist, from various vendors [e.g. Galileos (Sirona, Germany), MedView (Italy)]. This provides the clinician with the opportunity to use chair-side image display, real-time analysis and multiplanar rendering (MPR) modes that are task specific.[1] Because the CBCT volumetric data set is isotropic, the entire volume can be reoriented, so that the patient's anatomic features are realigned. In addition, cursor-driven measurement algorithms allow the clinician to do real-time dimensional assessment. With the improvement in the third party software, computer-aided design (CAD), computer-aided manufacturing (CAM) technology is also now integrated, thereby assisting the implantologist in designing the surgical guides and final prosthesis.

REDUCED IMAGE ARTIFACT

With manufacturers' artifact suppression algorithms and increasing number of projections, it has been shown that CBCT images can result in a low level of metal artifact, particularly in secondary reconstructions designed for viewing the teeth and jaws [metal artifact reduction software (MARS), Sirona].[1]

The CBCT imaging gives dentists the opportunity to diagnose and plan treatment more efficiently, and practically, can be used for everything—taking out a tooth that is close to the nerve, exposing a tooth for orthodontics, for implants, temporomandibular joint (TMJ) treatment and trauma.

Three-dimensional imaging touches all aspects of dentistry, from endodontics looking at teeth cross-sectionally to orthodontics.

In implant treatment planning, even for simple cases, cone beam imaging allows for concise and predictable treatment planning. Anatomic landmarks such as foramina and the mandibular canal can be precisely marked and cross-sectional views accurately show the width and length of available bone, give indications to the thickness and density of the bone, and provide virtual implant placement of virtually all implants from software libraries. This philosophy has quickly expanded into all phases of our practice of dentistry. It is by no means implying that 3D images are required for all patients, but rather there are cases where 2Ds are simply not enough and the addition of the third dimension, when applicable—becomes the only means of providing an accurate diagnosis. The presence of this technology has forever altered the standard of care in our profession with respect to diagnosis and treatment planning. The 3D cone beam imaging has raised the bar and redefined the standard of care for many areas of dental practice. There is no denying that 3D diagnostic imaging will continue to dominate and influence clinical practice. The trend to obtain more accurate 3D data with less 'guesswork' will undoubtedly lead us to better treatment planning decisions and hopefully more predictable outcomes.

To say it with George Bernard Shaw's words, "Progress is impossible without change and those who cannot change their minds cannot change anything".

REFERENCES

1. Scarfe WC, Farman AG, Sukovic P. Clinical applications of cone-beam computed tomography in dental practice. J Can Dent Assoc. 2006;72(1):75-80.
2. Cohnen M, Kemper J, Möbes O, et al. Radiation dose in dental radiology. Eur Radiol. 2002;12(3):634-7.
3. Schulze D, Heiland M, Thurmann H, et al. Radiation exposure during midfacial imaging using 4- and 16-slice computed tomography, cone beam computed tomography systems and conventional radiography. Dentomaxillofac Radiol. 2004;33(2):83–6.
4. Heiland M, Schulze D, Rother U, et al. Postoperative imaging of zygomaticomaxillary complex fractures using digital volume tomography. J Oral Maxillofac Surg. 2004;62(11):1387-91.
5. Mah JK, Danforth RA, Bumann A, et al. Radiation absorbed in maxillofacial imaging with a new dental computed tomography device. Oral Surg Oral Med Oral Pathol Oral Radiol Endod. 2003;96(4):508-13.
6. Ludlow JB, Davies-Ludlow LE, Brooks SL. Dosimetry of two extraoral direct digital imaging devices: NewTom cone beam CT and Orthophos Plus DS panoramic unit. Dentomaxillofac Radiol. 2003;32(4):229-34.

4 Chapter

Anatomical Landmarks on Cone Beam Computed Tomography

Sushma P Jaju

INTRODUCTION

Humans can diagnose pathology, when they understand normal structures.

Dentists and specialists worldwide are trained efficiently in diagnosis using traditional imaging modalities like intraoral and panoramic radiography. These imaging modalities have been taught for decades now in dental schools and in continuing dental education programs.

The main hurdle in understanding the images formed by cone beam computed tomography (CBCT) is lack of familiarity of oral maxillofacial specialists with the concept of three-dimensional (3D) imaging. Understanding the various images in different planes requires high level of competency, which is currently limited to fewer individuals.[1]

Diagnosis of maxillofacial pathology is only possible once you identify the normal anatomical structures. This Chapter looks into the various anatomical landmarks relevant to dental specialists as observed on various planes, i.e. sagittal, coronal and axial.

VISUALIZATION OF CBCT IMAGES

Imagine patient sitting in front of you on the dental chair. Just as his/her right side is the opposite side of the dentist, similarly, while viewing the CBCT images either on computer screen or film viewer, structures identified on the dentist's right side would represent the anatomical structures on the patient's left and vice versa.

Most of the CBCT manufacturers have labeled images with right and left sides or buccal/lingual/palatal/oral on the images, thus easing the procedure of identification (Figs 4.1A to E).

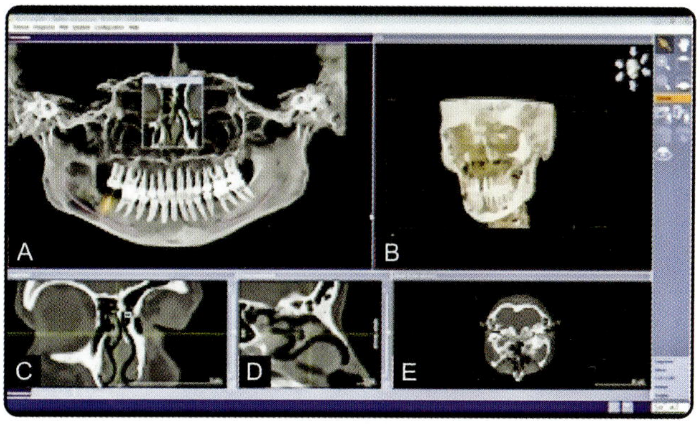

Figures 4.1A to E: Side identification present on various screen for easy orientation

MAXILLARY LANDMARKS

Nasopalatine Foramen/Incisive Foramen

The nasopalatine canal is usually described as being located in the midline of the palate, posterior to the central maxillary incisors.[2] The canal divides into two canaliculi on its way to the nasal cavity and terminates at the nasal floor with an opening (known as the foramina of Stenson) at either side of the septum. The canal contains the nasopalatine (incisive) nerve and the terminal branch of the descending nasopalatine artery, as well as fibrous connective tissue, fat and even small salivary glands.[2] On a periapical radiograph, it appears as a round to oval radiolucency between the roots and in the region of the middle and apical third of the central incisors (Fig. 4.2).[3]

The radiographic appearance varies depending upon the anatomical variations and also technique variation. On the CBCT, nasopalatine canal can be visualized as a canal starting from the floor of nasal cavity with dual foramina and exiting through the incisive foramen and spreading to anterior aspect of the hard palate (Figs 4.3 to 4.5).

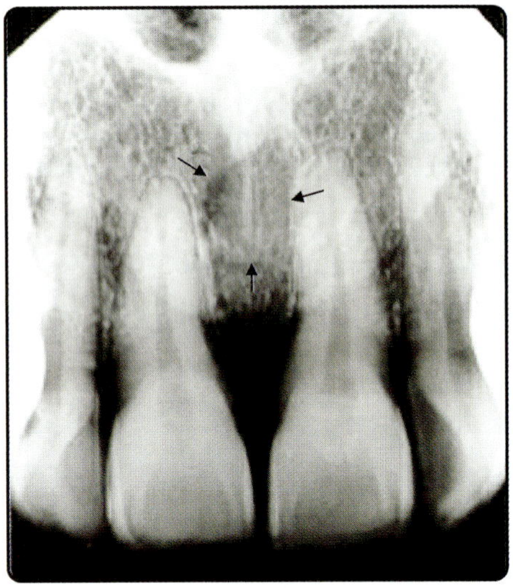

Figure 4.2: Intraoral periapical radiograph of maxillary central incisor showing nasopalatine canal between central incisors

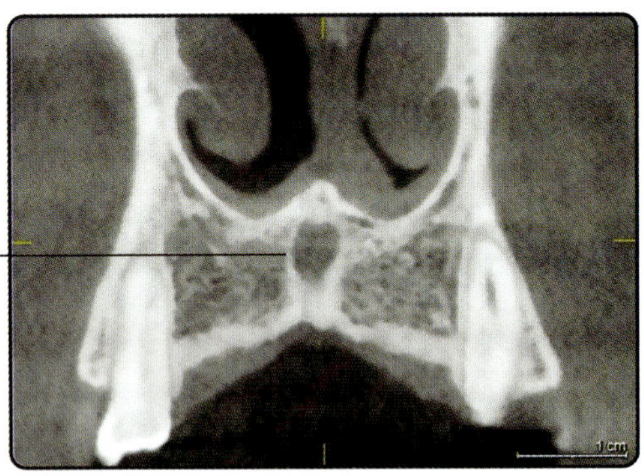

Figure 4.3: Coronal view showing incisive foramen

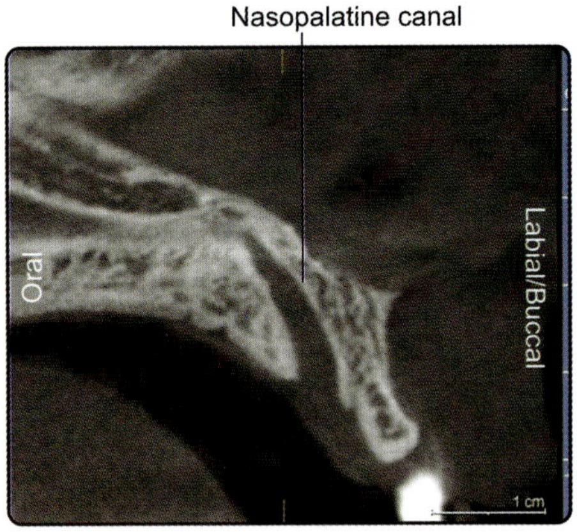

Figure 4.4: Cross-sectional view showing entire length of nasopalatine canal

Dental esthetics has become an important issue in implant dentistry. In the anterior maxilla, patients consider the esthetic outcome to be an essential factor, often surpassing even functional aspects of the dental implant therapy.[2] Implant contact with neural tissue may result in failure of osseointegration or lead to sensory dysfunction like paresthesia or numbness.[2] In view of these potential complications, the morphology and dimensions of the nasopalatine canal should be properly evaluated before placement of dental implants in the vicinity of this anatomical structures (Fig. 4.6).

On CBCT images, anatomical variations of nasopalatine canal can be seen. These canals are best visualized on coronal images. Type A, a single canal; Type B, two parallel canals; Type C, variations of the Y type of canal with one oral/palatal opening (one-fourth incisive foramen) and two or more nasal openings (one-fourth foramina of Stenson)[2] (Figs 4.7 to 4.9).

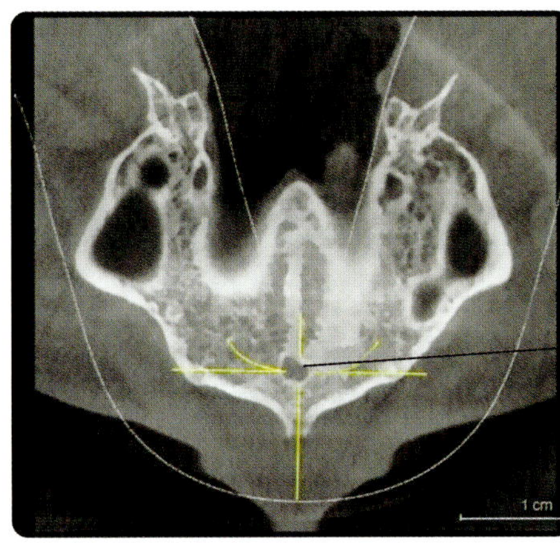

Figure 4.5: Axial view showing incisive foramen in anterior region of hard palate

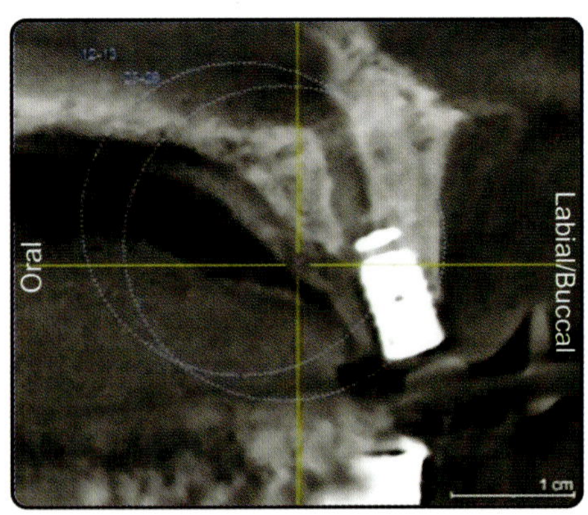

Figure 4.6: Cross-sectional view showing implant placed on nasopalatine canal

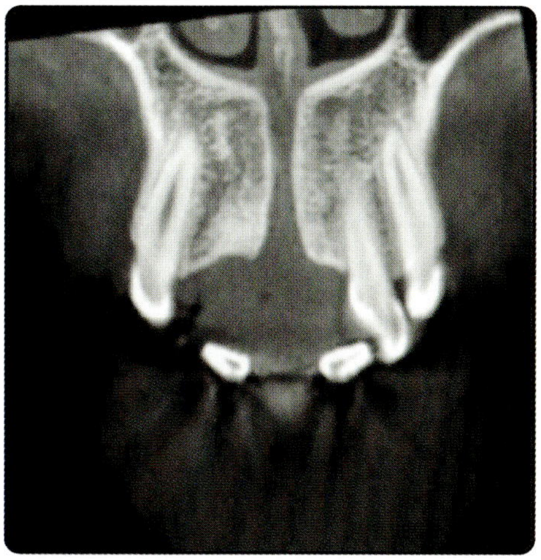

Figure 4.7: Type A nasopalatine canal

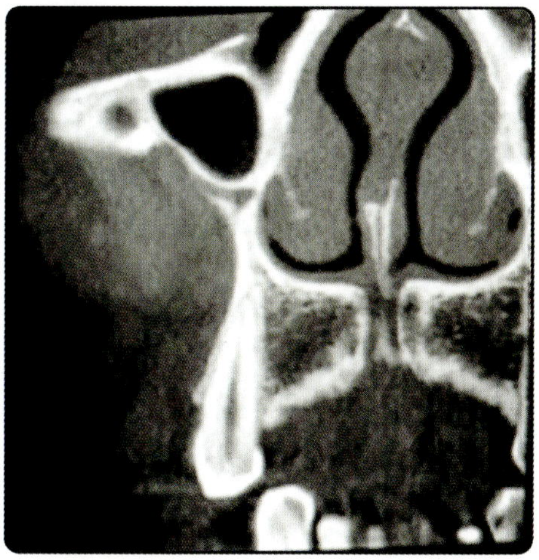

Figure 4.8: Type B nasopalatine canal

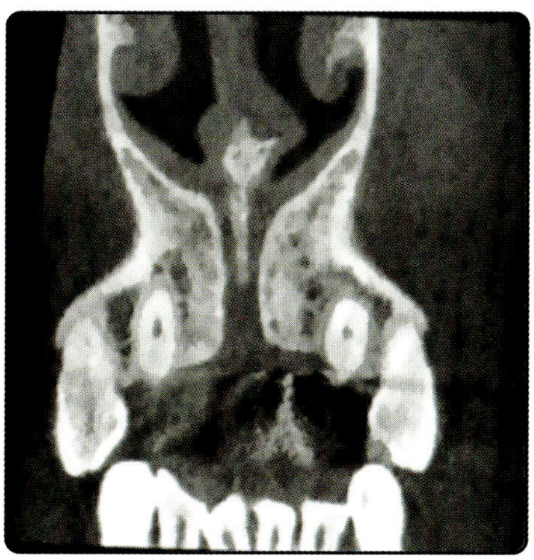

Figure 4.9: Type C nasopalatine canal

Gender variations in appearance of nasopalatine canal were present in the study done by Jacob et al.[2] In their study, male patients had a significantly increased length of the nasopalatine canal and higher values for the three different buccal bone plate measurements than females. Age significantly influenced the length of the nasopalatine canal with a decrease of the mean value in older patients.

Contradictory results were present with respect to width of crestal buccal bone wall with respect to duration of edentulism. In study conducted by Mardinger et al, the buccal bone plate anterior to the canal lost about 60% of its mean width when comparing fully dentate patients with edentulous ridges.[2] In contrast, Jacobs et al reported an increase in the canal diameter and foramina (nasopalatine foramina and incisive foramen) with the degree of ridge resorption accompanied by edentulism. The differences in the findings of the two studies could originate in the fact that only partially edentulous patients (not fully edentulous) were included in the present study and the average age of the included patients was 43.09 years (in contrast to 58.12 years in the study by Mardinger et al, 2008).[2]

Nasal Cavities

Nasal cavities (nasal fossa) are air-filled cavities, appearing as a radiolucent shadow on the periapical radiograph of maxillary central incisors. Intraoral periapical radiograph shows only the floor of nasal cavity. The CBCT shows entire dimension of nasal cavity as a radiolucent shadow. Coronal views are best to demonstrate the nasal cavity structures and paranasal sinuses.[1] The nasal septum is identified as radiopaque, partially ossified structures in the midline, dividing nasal cavity into two fossa. Deviated nasal septum is easily identifiable on CBCT coronal image. Inferior nasal concha is an independent facial bone, whereas middle and superior nasal conchae are parts of ethmoid bone. Middle nasal conchae are two of the osseous processes that separate nasal cavities into meatus or turbinates. The two well-defined and well-corticated soft tissue content structures in the anterolateral wall of the nasal cavity bilaterally are identified as nasolacrimal ducts. The nasolacrimal ducts drain tears from the orbits to the inferior nasal turbinates (Figs 4.10 to 4.13).

In cases of placement of maxillary anterior implant, the identification of this anatomical structure is important to prevent postoperative complications. The CBCT allows accurate measurement of the ridge height from the crest of the ridge to the floor of nasal cavity. Ideally, the implant length should be 2 mm away from the anatomical structure. Nasal cavity appears as a radiolucent shadow, seen on consecutive sections of cross-sectional images, thus assisting in identification of any pathologies of nasal cavity.[3]

Maxillary Sinus

Maxillary sinus is a critical anatomical structure in the maxillary posterior region of the jaw. The maxillary sinus, like the other paranasal sinuses, is an air-containing cavity lined with mucous membrane. It develops by the invagination of mucous membrane from the nasal cavity. Being the largest of the paranasal sinuses, it normally occupies virtually the entire body of the maxilla. The maxillary sinus is a pyramidal shaped cavity. Healthy sinus appears as a radiolucent (black) shadow because of the fact that air attenuates X-rays minimally. The maxillary sinuses are often asymmetric. Likewise, the anterior sinus borders are important in the anterior posterior implants, especially in cases of severe maxillary anterior ridge resorption.[3]

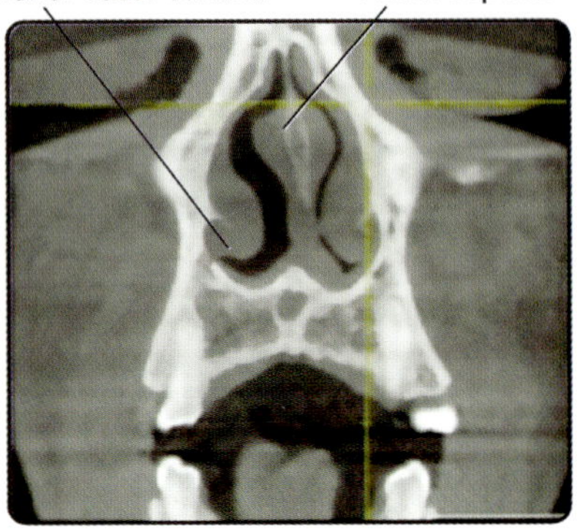

Figure 4.10: Coronal section at the level of canine region

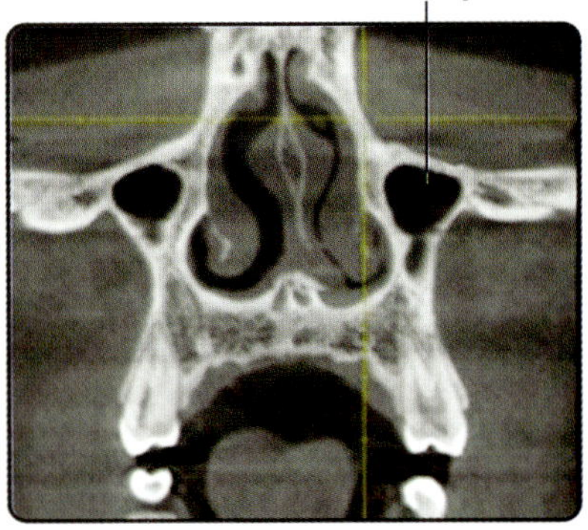

Figure 4.11: Coronal section of nasal cavity at premolar level

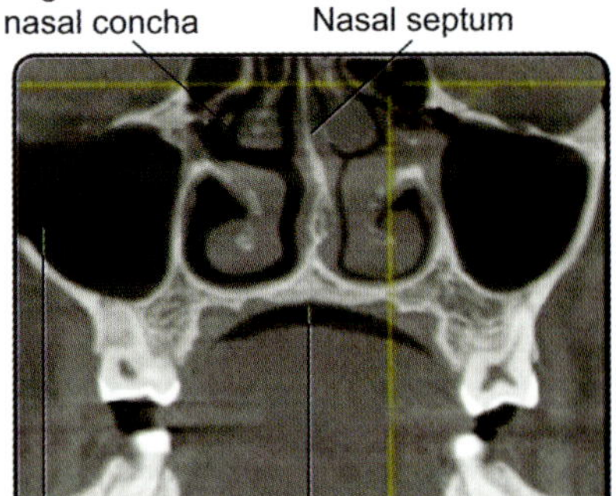

Figure 4.12: Coronal section of nasal cavity at molar region

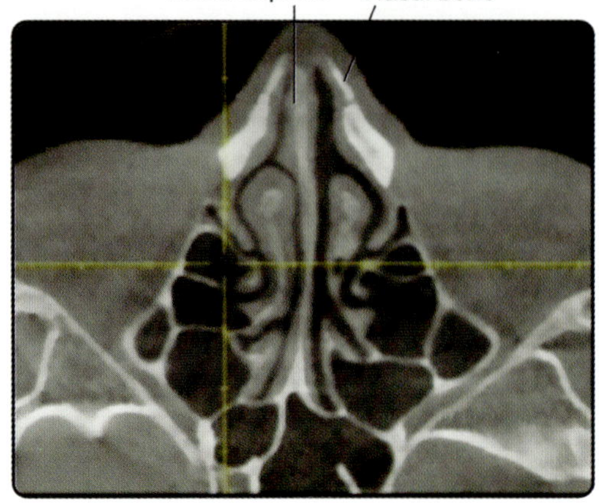

Figure 4.13: Axial view showing nasal cavity

In conventional imaging techniques, entire sinus cannot be visualized in a single film, but on CBCT images maxillary sinus can be viewed in various sections simultaneously. Pathoses appeared as mucosal thickening and diagnosed preoperatively, treatment could be provided prior to implant placement. The CBCT provides information regarding the cortical bone in the floor of the nasal cavity and maxillary sinuses prior to implant placement. Coronal view at the level of anterior third of the orbit shows the draining sites of maxillary sinuses. These are narrow passages toward the superomedial wall of the maxillary sinuses leading into the middle nasal turbinate. Osteomeatal complex is formed partially from the ethmoid bone and a thin pointy osseous process on the antral wall of the nasal cavity known as uncinate process. Blockage of osteomeatal complex results in accumulation of inflammatory products into the sinus. Identification of these pathology is important prior to sinus grafting procedures (Figs 4.14 to 4.16).[1]

Lana JP et al in their study on anatomic variations in maxillary sinus by CBCT detected pneumatization (83.2%), antral septa (44.4%), hypoplasia (4.8%) and exostosis (2.6%). The identified lesions were mucosal thickening (≤ 3 mm in 54.8% and > 3 mm in 62.6%), polypoid lesions (21.4%), discontinuity of the sinus floor (17.4%), air-fluid level (4.4%), bone thickening of the maxillary sinus wall (3.8%), antroliths (3.2%), discontinuity of the sinus lateral wall (2.6%), sinus opacification (1.8%) and foreign body (1.6%).[4] This highlights the important role, the CBCT plays in understanding and diagnosing maxillary sinus pathologies.

A deep depression on the lateral wall of nasopharynx bilaterally as seen on axial images showing eustachian tube, which communicates between inner and external ear. Just posterior to the eustachian tube separated by soft tissue projection, lies the pharyngeal recess or fossa of Rosenmüller (Figs 4.17 to 4.19).[1]

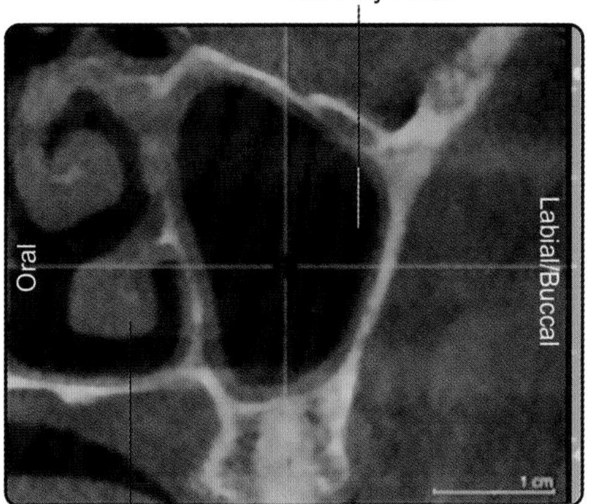

Figure 4.14: Coronal view of maxillary sinus showing floor, medial, lateral and roof

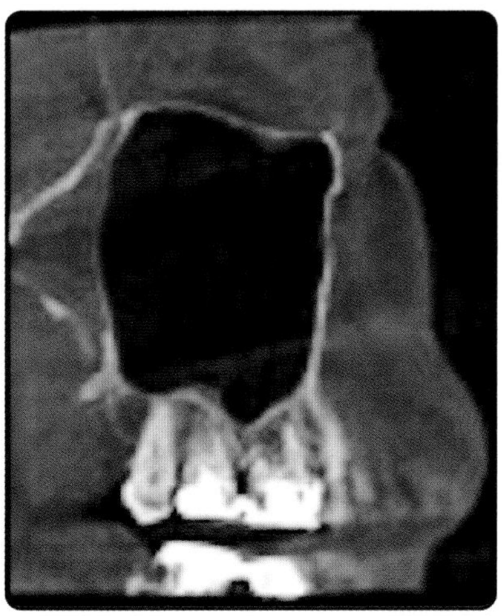

Figure 4.15: Sagittal view of the healthy maxillary sinus showing anterior and posterior wall

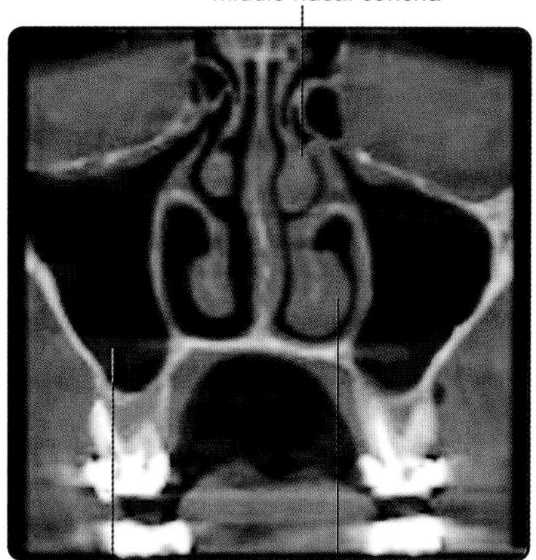

Figure 4.16: Coronal view of the both healthy maxillary sinuses appearing as radiolucent shadow

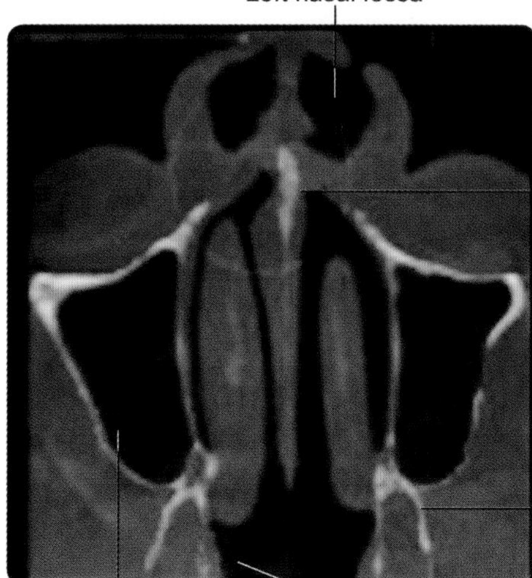

Figure 4.17: Axial view of both the maxillary sinuses

Greater and Lesser Palatine Foramen

The anatomy of the greater palatine canal is of interest to dentists, oral maxillofacial surgeons and otolaryngologists performing procedures in this area (e.g. administration of local anesthesia, dental implant placement, orthognathic Le Fort I osteotomies and sinonasal surgeries).[5] It houses

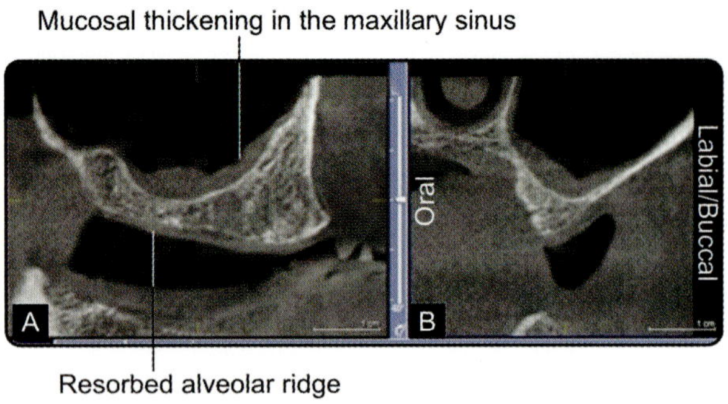

Figures 4.18A and B: Sagittal and cross-sectional window showing mucosal thickening in the floor of maxillary sinus

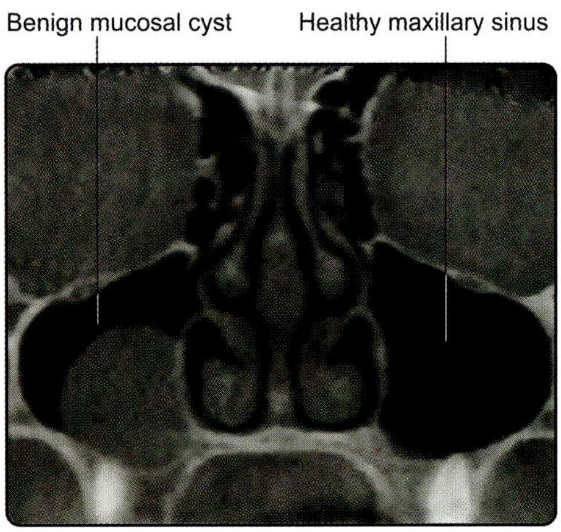

Figure 4.19: Benign mucosal cyst in right maxillary sinus; left maxillary sinus appears normal

the descending palatine artery (a branch of the third division of the maxillary artery), and greater and lesser palatine nerves (branches of the maxillary division of the trigeminal nerve) and their posterior, inferior, lateral nasal branches. These vessels run on the hard palate from posterior to anterior, just superior to the palatal roots of the maxillary molars in soft tissue in a palatal mucosa.[5]

The walls of the greater palatine canal are formed anteriorly by the infratemporal surface of the maxilla, posteriorly by the pterygoid process of the sphenoid, and medially by the perpendicular plate of the palatine.[6] The maxillary sinus is located anterior, and the nasal cavity and concha medial and the pterygoid plates posterior to the greater palatine canal. The anatomy of these structures undoubtedly affects the anatomy of the greater palatine canal due to their proximal relationships. When performing surgical procedures in this area, preservation of the descending palatine artery and palatine nerves is essential to avoid excessive bleeding and to maintain nerve supply to the maxilla.[5] In other cases, regional nerve block may be unsuccessful if excessive resistance is met when injecting local anesthesia into the greater palatine canal, presumably the result of anatomic variation. The CBCT clearly demonstrates the greater and lesser palatine foramina on axial views (Figs 4.20 to 4.25). The average length of the canal is found to be 29 mm with a range of 22–40 mm.[5]

Ethmoid and Sphenoid Sinuses

The ethmoid sinuses are made up of numerous, small, thin-walled air cells separated by the vomer bone in the midline. Their complicated anatomy gave them the characterization of the ethmoid labyrinth. The sphenoid sinus is located just posterior to the ethmoid sinuses. These are air cavities that are irregular in shape and size, located just

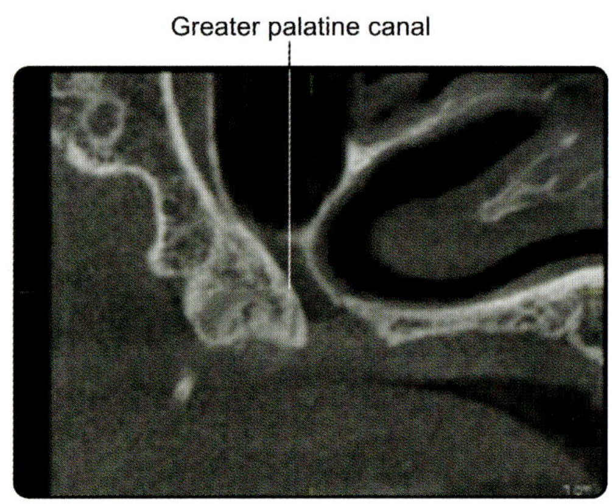

Figure 4.20: Tangential view of greater palatine canal extending anteroinferiorly

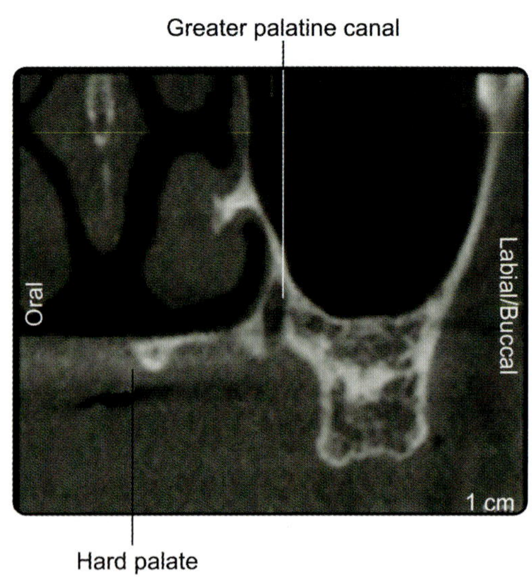

Figure 4.21: Coronal view showing greater palatine canal

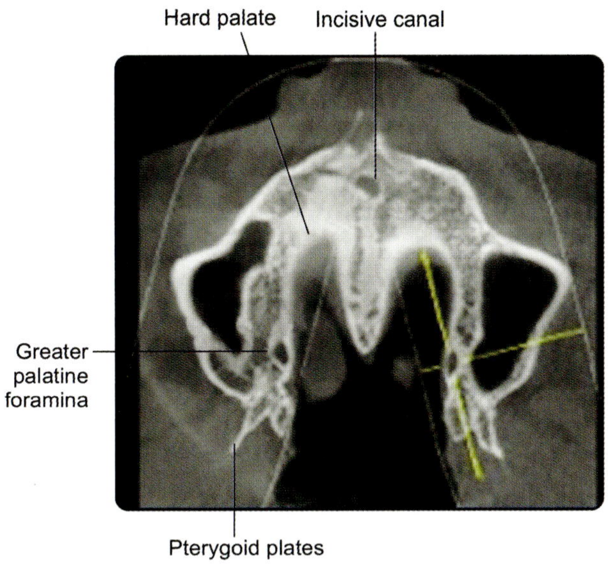

Figure 4.22: Axial view showing greater and lesser palatine foramina

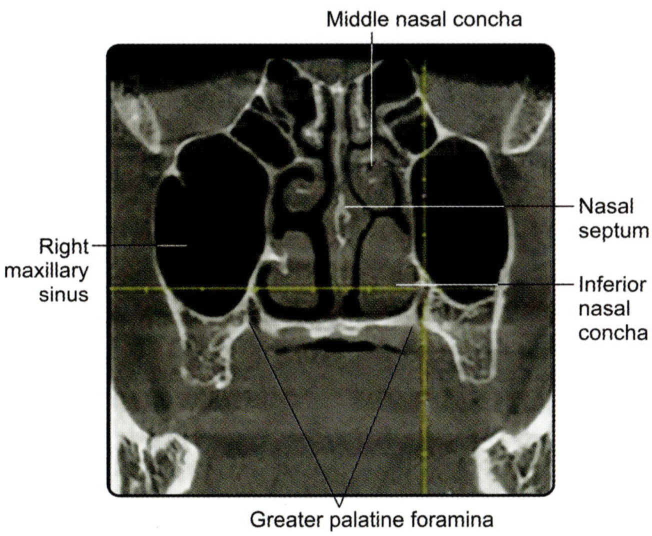

Figure 4.23: Coronal view showing right and left greater palatine canals

below the base of sphenoid bone. Anatomic variation and septations are often present. Healthy sinuses appears as a radiolucent shadow (Fig. 4.26).[1]

Frontal Sinus

Frontal sinus is one of the paranasal sinuses, which is present on the frontal part of the skull. Coronal view at the level of anterior part of the orbit reveals entire anatomy of the frontal sinus. Anterior and posterior recess have been

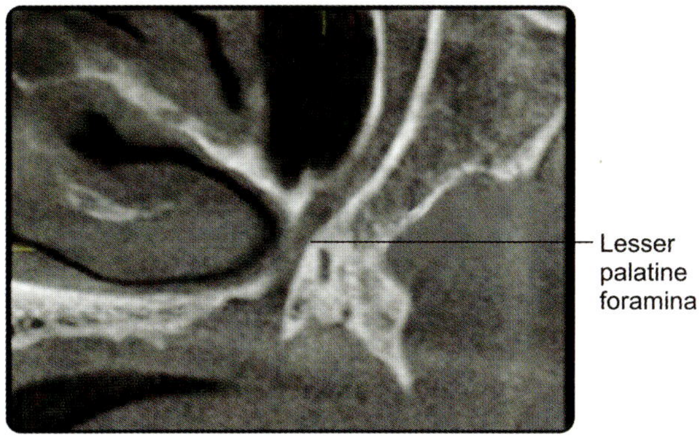

Figure 4.24: Tangential view of lesser palatine canal

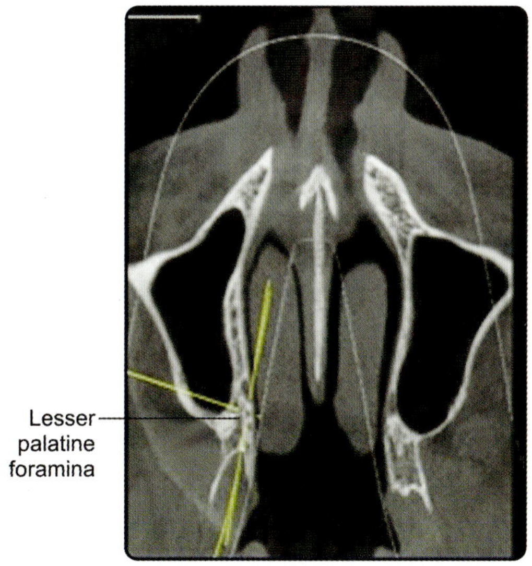

Figure 4.25: Axial view showing greater and lesser palatine foramina

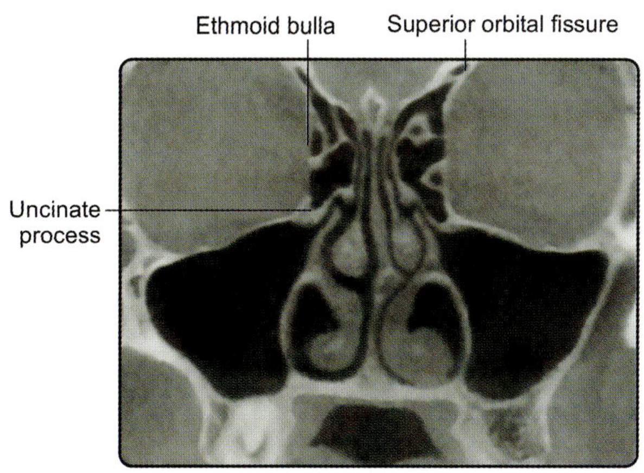

Figure 4.26: Coronal view showing ethmoid sinuses

clearly identified on CBCT images. As mentioned earlier, healthy frontal sinus appears as a radiolucent image; whereas in conditions such as sinusitis, mucosal thickening or grayish shadow is evident (Fig. 4.27).

Hard Palate and Soft Palate

The hard palate is a thin horizontal bony plate of the skull, located in the roof of the mouth. It spans the arch formed by the upper teeth. It is formed by the palatine process of the maxilla and horizontal plate of palatine bone. It forms a partition between the nasal passages and the mouth. Hard palate appears as a thick radiopaque shadow above the apices of maxillary teeth separating oral cavity and nasal cavity. Posteriorly, hard palate continues as soft palate. Soft palate forms the posterior part of the root of the oral cavity. Soft palate is seen as a grayish horizontal shadow extending from distal aspect of hard palate and sloping backwards and downwards. It is distinguished from hard palate, as it does not contain bone (Fig. 4.28).

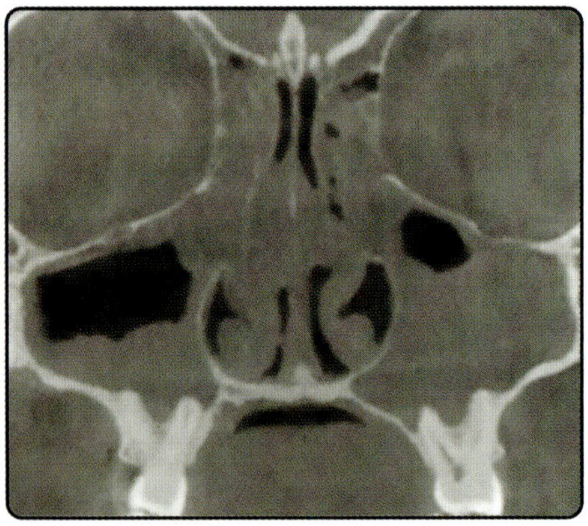

Figure 4.27: Coronal view showing pansinusitis

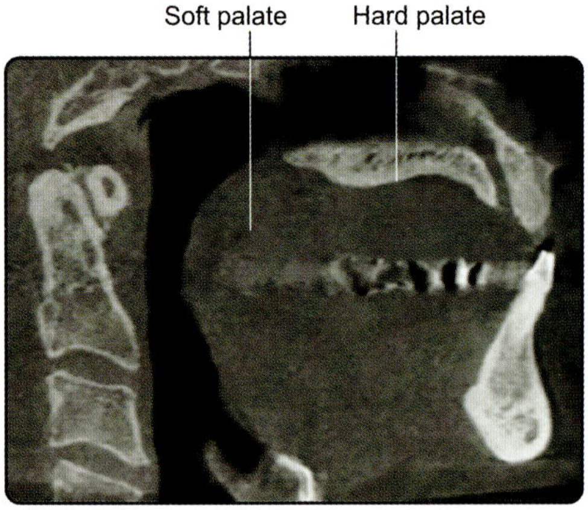

Figure 4.28: Sagittal view showing hard and soft palate

Zygomatic Arch

The zygomatic arch or cheek bone is formed by the zygomatic process of temporal bone (a bone extending forward from the side of the skull, over the opening of the ear) and the temporal process of the zygomatic bone (the side of the cheekbone), the two being united by an oblique suture (zygomaticotemporal suture) (Figs 4.29 to 4.31).

Zygomatic arch is commonly involved in zygomatic complex fracture. Two-dimensional imaging like posteroanterior (PA) Water's view shows the level of fracture line, but amount of displacement of fracture fragment is not depicted clearly. The CBCT shows zygomatic arch as a thick radiopaque shadow on lateral aspect of maxilla. Axial view is best view to demonstrate the extent and location of fracture (Fig. 4.32).

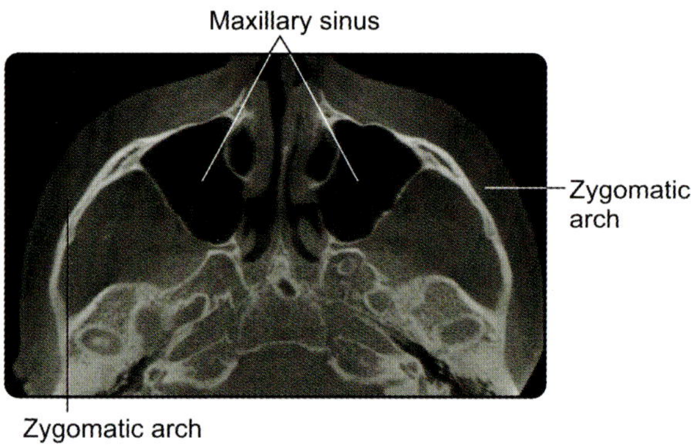

Figure 4.29: Axial view showing bilateral normal zygomatic arches

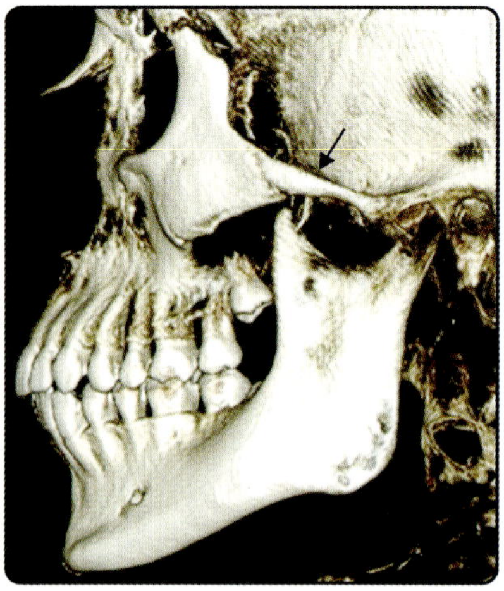

Figure 4.30: Three-dimensional reconstruction showing normal left zygomatic arch

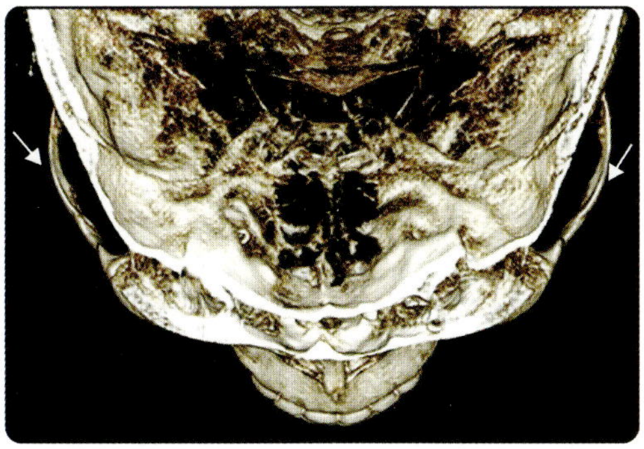

Figure 4.31: Axial three-dimensional reconstructed view showing bilateral zygomatic arch

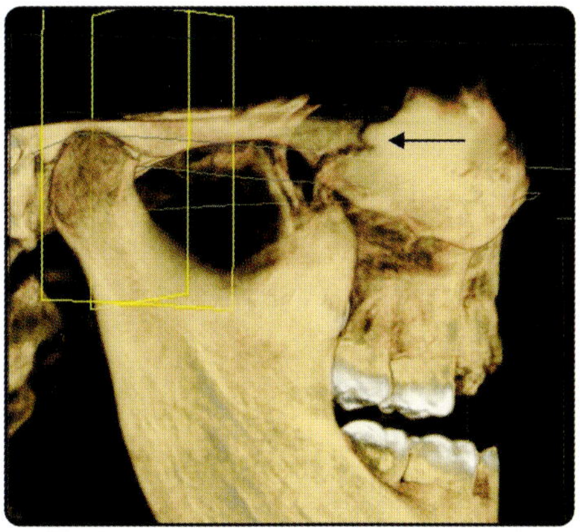

Figure 4.32: Right zygomatic arch fracture seen on three-dimensional reconstruction

MANDIBULAR LANDMARKS

Lingual Vascular Foramen

Mandibular interforaminal region (premolar-premolar) was considered to be the safest zone for implant placement. But recent literature suggests that it is no longer considered to be the risk-free zone for implants. A significant anatomic structure in the lingual aspect of the mandibular bone, along the midline of the mandible is the lingual foramen or foramina, which harbors terminal branches of lingual artery. These are closely associated with genial tubercles, which serve as muscle attachment. Ennis, Suzuki and Sakai, McDonnell et al Darriba and Mendonca- Caridad and Givol et al assumed a vascular content being an anastomosis of the sublingual branch of right and left lingual arteries.[3]

The diameter of these canals are related to the blood-supplying capacity of the blood vessel, and as a result, if they are wide enough, they may bleed significantly if injured during implant surgery resulting in sublingual hematoma formation, asphyxia and death. Depending upon the amount of residual ridge resorption, these canals may be seen close to the crest of the ridge. Goaz and White stated that the foramen and canal were the termination of the incisive branch of the mandibular canal. According to Yoshida et al found low frequency of occurrence (45.7%) of lingual foramen on internal surface of mandible on dry cadavers. According to McDonnell et al, lingual foramen was present in 99.04% in midline of mandible. These canals run from lingual cortical plate extending inferiorly toward the cancellous part of bone. Cross-sectional images on CBCT are ideal for locating these canals. Occasionally, double lingual vascular canals can also be seen. Yoshida et al believed that lingual artery visualization on radiography was difficult and CT provides an adequate visualization of the vascular canal.[3] Multiplanar reformation (MPR) provide excellent visualization of midline mandibular structure clearly depicting the lingual canal and size of the lingual canals correlate well with the results of anatomic studies.[1]

The small difference in the size values of the canals can probably be attributed to the fact that the smallest canals were too small to be visible because of the limited resolution capability of CT. Gultekin et al in their study revealed typical lingual canal locations were the middle of the mandible and the premolar regions (Figs 4.33A to E and 4.34A and B).

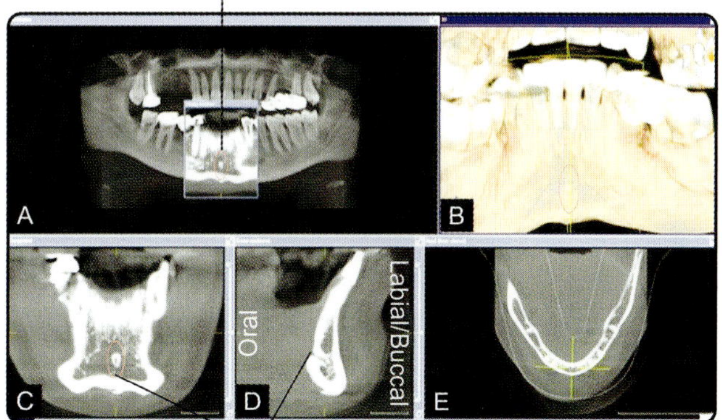

Figures 4.33A to E: Lingual vascular canal in various slices present at midline of mandible

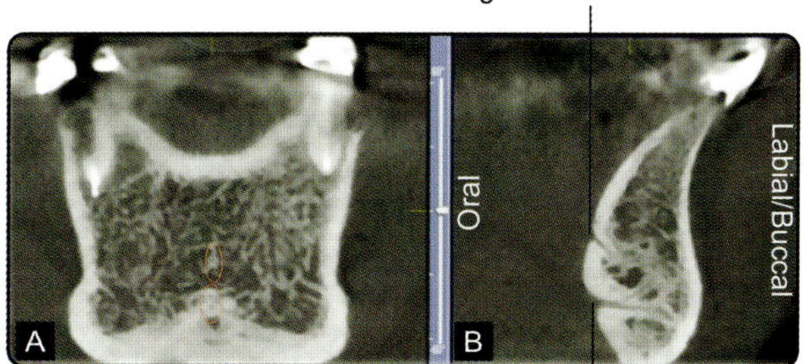

Figures 4.34A and B: Double lingual vascular foramina

Mental Foramen

Mandibular nerve exists through the mental foramen. It transmits mental nerve, artery and vein. Mental nerve is a branch of inferior alveolar nerve, which supplies sensation to lower lip and the labial mucosa and lower canines and premolars.[7]

Intraoral periapical (IOPA) radiographs shows either a slit shaped or a complete dimension of the mental foramen depending upon the angulation of the X-ray beam to the mental foramen.

Cone beam CT is the radiographic method of choice to depict mental foramen. Variations in the position of the mental foramen are also common. Typically, the foramen is located halfway between the alveolar crest and the lower mandibular border between the first and second premolars (Fig. 4.35).

However, it may be found as far anterior as the canine and as far posterior as the first and second molars. The neurovascular bundle may loop downward, forward and medially before exiting from the foramen in a posterosuperior direction. In older edentulous individuals with resorbed ridges, the foramen may be near or may actually emerge from the alveolar crest likewise (Figs 4.36 and 4.37).

Accessory mental foramina is also a common finding with an overall incidence of 6%–10%. The accessory mental foramen (AMF) was defined as a buccal foramen with continuity to the mandibular canal. Also, a buccal foramen showing continuity without mandibular canal was considered to be nutrient foramen. The incidence of accessory mental foramen varies between ethnic groups and is reported as follows:[7]

- 2.6% in French
- 1.4% in American Whites
- 5.7% in American Blacks
- 3.3% in Greeks
- 1.5% in Russians
- 3.0% in Hungarians.

Gershenson et al in a study of 525 dry mandibles and 50 cadavers, reported incidences of 23 mandibles with double foramina (4.3%), four with triple foramina (0.7%) and one skull with four foramina on one side.[8] The absence and variation of accessory mental foramina has been reported in dry human mandibles and radiographs previously, and can range from 0.2% to 10.6% on one side.[8] The presence of more than one MF, referred to as accessory mental foramina (AMF), has been noted on dissection, surgical findings, conventional radiographs, spiral CT and CBCT.[8]

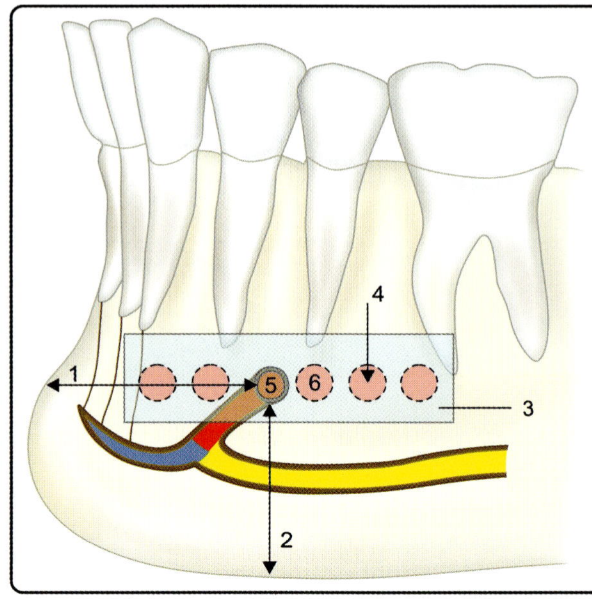

Figure 4.35: Anatomical variations of the mental foramen (MF) position in the horizontal plane in relation to the roots of teeth; blue, mandibular incisive canal (MIC); red, mental canal (the anterior opening of the mandibular canal); yellow, mandibular canal. **1.** Distance from MF to midline of the mandible (approximate distance 28 mm); **2.** Distance from MF to the inferior border of the mandible (14–15 mm); **3.** Possible MF location zone in the horizontal plane in relation to the roots of teeth; **4.** The shape of MF can be round or oval, the diameter is 1.68–3.5 mm; **5.** Prevalence location of MF in the horizontal plane for Caucasian population; **6.** Prevalence location of MF in the horizontal plane for Mongoloids and African people. *Courtesy:* www.ejomr.org/JOMR/archives/2010/1/e3/e3ht.htm.

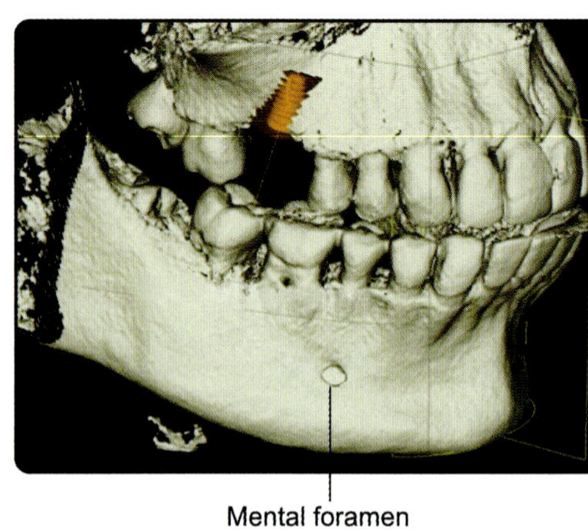

Figure 4.36: Mental foramen on three-dimensional reconstruction

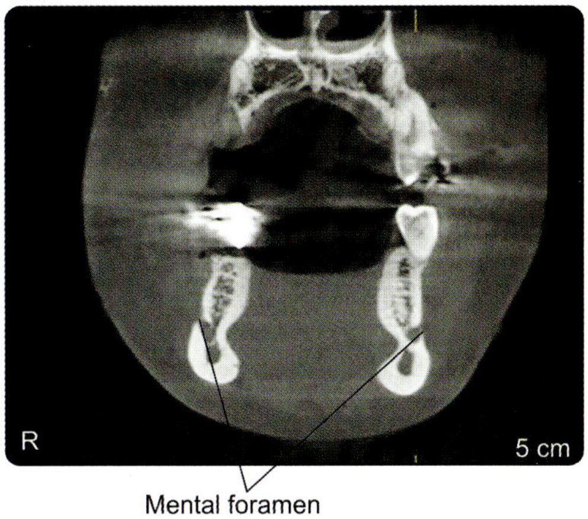

Figure 4.37: Coronal view showing bilateral mental foramen

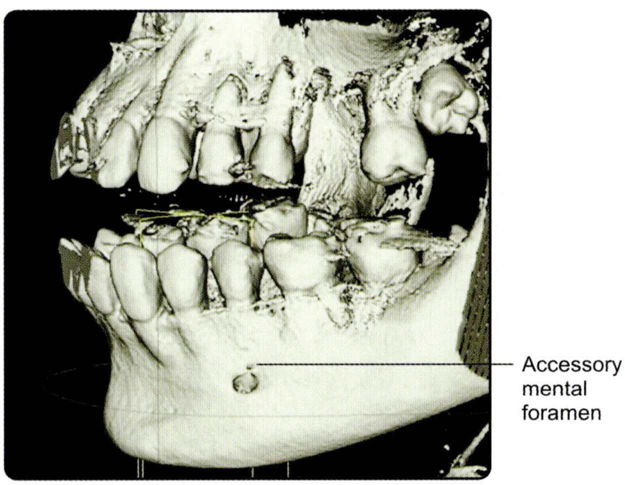

Figure 4.38: Three-dimensional construction showing accessory mental foramina superior to mental foramen

The AMF can be rarely observed with intraoral and panoramic radiography because the size is generally less than 1.0 mm.[8] The CT is the most accurate imaging modality for the identification and localization of the mandibular foramen, mandibular canal and MF. The localization of such structures, as well as their eventual anatomical variations, is of fundamental importance prior to any surgical and anesthetic procedure.[8] Result in study showed that incidence of accessory mental foramen in Indian population was 8.4%. Highest incidences of AMFs are reported in Negros and Maori mandibles. Position of the accessory mental foramina may be superior, inferior, anterior or posteriorly to mental foramen (Figs 4.38 to 4.41).

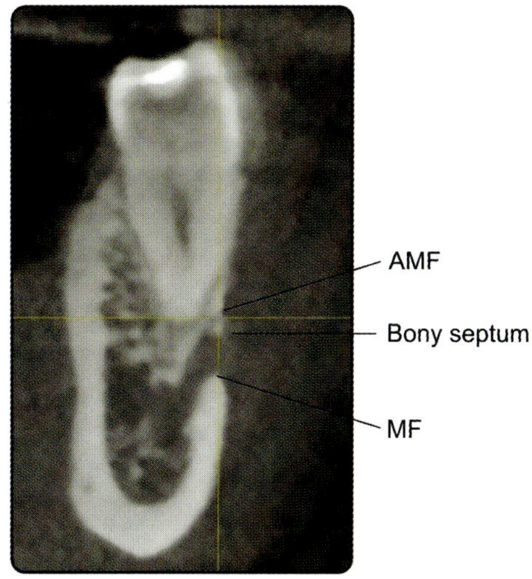

Figure 4.39: Cross-sectional and three-dimensional reconstruction of accessory mental foramina (AMF); mental foramen (MF)

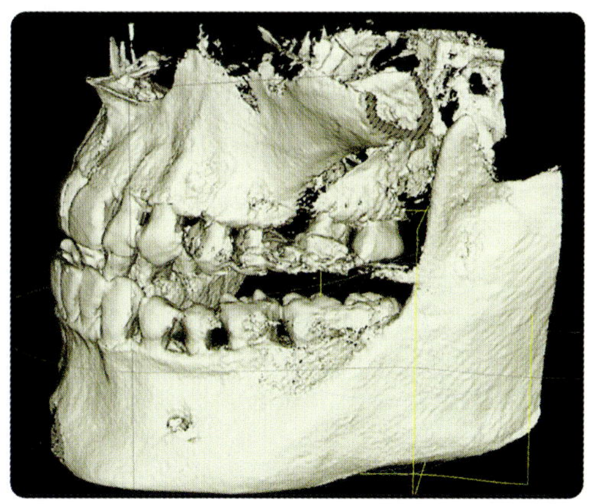

Figure 4.40: Accessory mental foramina inferior to mental foramen

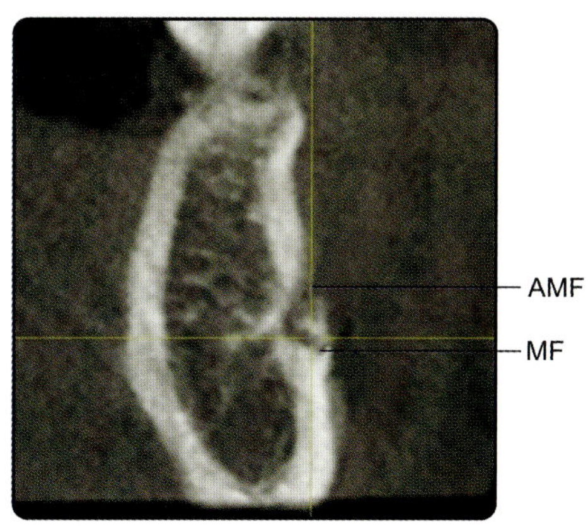

Figure 4.41: Cross-sectional image showing accessory mental foramina (AMF) below mental foramen (MF)

Anterior Loop of Mental Nerve

The final part of the inferior alveolar nerve sometimes passes below the lower border and the anterior wall of the mental foramen. After giving off the smaller mandibular incisive branch, the main branch curves back to enter the foramen and emerge to the soft tissues as the mental nerve. The section of the nerve in front of the mental foramen and just before its ramification to the incisive nerve can be defined as the anterior loop of the inferior alveolar nerve. Elective surgery in the area of the anterior mandible such as implant installation in the interforaminal region or symphysis bone harvesting, may violate the anterior loop resulting in neurosensory disturbances in the area of the lower lip and chin.[7]

This structure has a high prevalence (61.5%–96%) in cadaveric studies, with symmetric occurrence a common finding (76.2%), anterior loops were most often observed bilaterally, followed by on the right side only. The visibility of anterior loop reduces as the age of the subjects increased.[7] On consecutive cross-sectional images, round radiolucent shadow is appreciated anterior to mental foramina. These shadows represent anterior loop of mental nerve (refer Fig. 4.35).[3]

Mandibular Canal

Mandibular canal is the most critical anatomical structure in mandibular posterior region. Identification of this landmark is of prime importance prior to implant surgery, third molar disimpaction or periapical surgery. Conventional imaging cannot show the complete extend of the MC. Buccopalatal orientation of the MC is not appreciated even on panoramic radiograph. Canal may not be visible on conventional radiographic methods; it is probably related to the fact that the inferior alveolar neurovascular bundle is not always surrounded by an ossified canal. The bony sheath seems to disappear anteriorly toward the MF. Similarly, in edentulous patients, the diameter of the artery is smaller compared to dentate patients, and hence the visibility of the canal may be affected. The mandibular nerve may course diagonally from a lingual location posterior to a buccal location in the area of the MF. The buccal-lingual position of the nerve can only be seen on CBCT—either axial or cross-sectional views of the mandibular ridges.[3] Cross-sectional slices provide consecutive sections, which depicts the course of the inferior alveolar nerve up to MF (Figs 4.42A and B).

Currently, all CBCT software have color coding by which MC can be color coded and traced entirely from lingual foramen till the MF (Fig. 4.43). This eases identification of the mandibular canal, which may be sometimes difficult on conventional imaging especially in osteoporotic individuals. Variation in anatomy of MC such as bifid mandibular canal, is also identified easily on CBCT (Figs 4.44A and B).

Cervical Spine

Sagittal images of the neck are best for assessment of the cervical spine and the airway. The cervical spine is only partially visualized in a CBCT scan (Figs 4.45 and 4.46). The normal appearance of the vertebral bodies include a fairly square body with thin cortical outline, a cancellous component of homogenous density and a fairly symmetric spacing between vertebrae visible in the scan.[1]

Airway Space

The airway is identified as an irregular shaped, elongated low-density area to cervical part of the vertebral column. The position of the epiglottis, laryngeal opening below the epiglottis and the position of the tongue may have an effect on the diameter of the airway. The CBCT is the ideal imaging techniques to evaluate patients with sleep apnea by

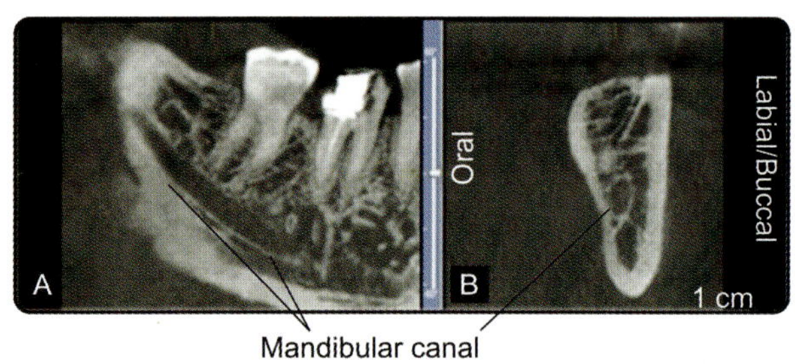

Figures 4.42A and B: Mandibular canal. **A.** Mandibular canal seen on tangential image as linear canal below apices of teeth; **B.** Cross-sectional image shows a round radiolucent shadow close to lingual cortical plate.

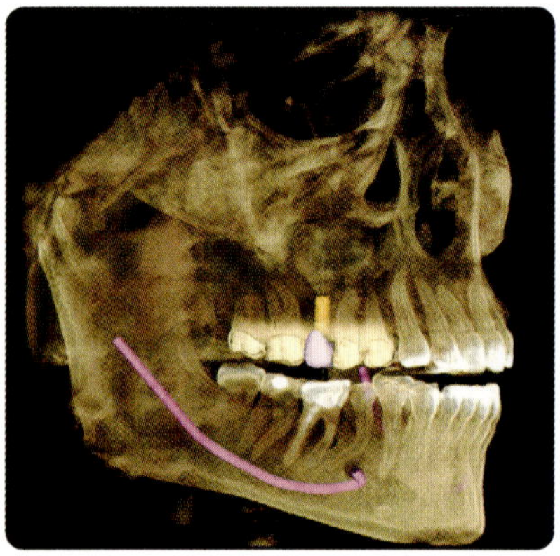

Figure 4.43: Color coding of mandibular canal

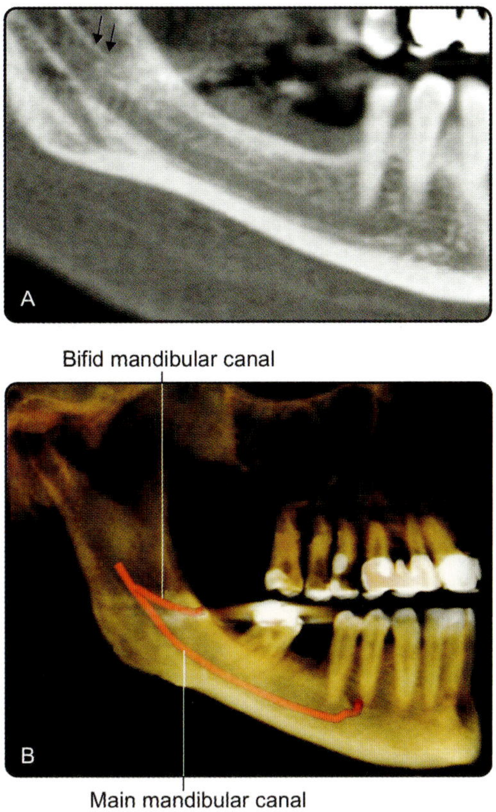

Figures 4.44A and B: Bifid mandibular canal (arrow marks)

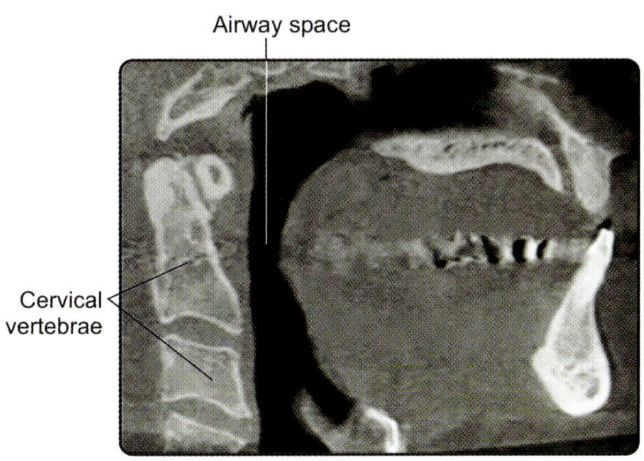

Figure 4.45: Sagittal images showing cervical spine

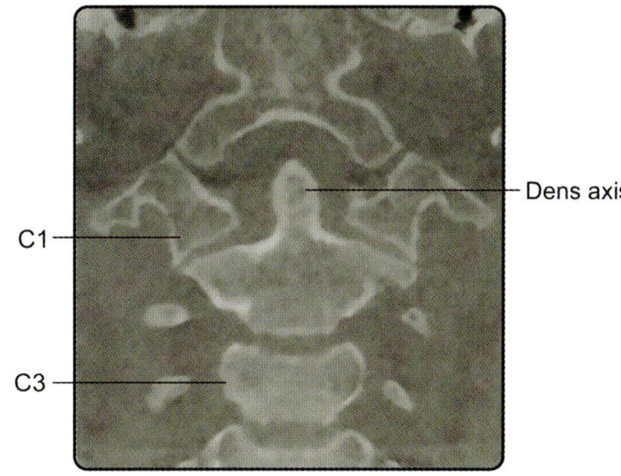

Figure 4.46: Coronal view showing the cervical spine

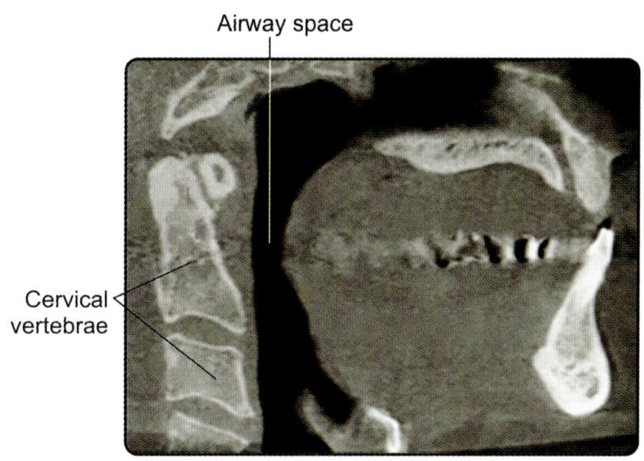

Figure 4.47: Airway space on sagittal image

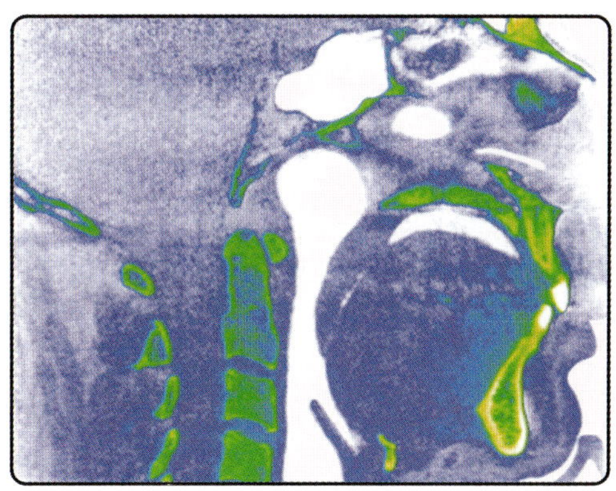

Figure 4.48: Volumetric reconstruction showing airway space and vertebral column

analyzing the air space. The CBCT is suited to aiding our understanding of the upper airway; all of the intricacies are visible and not hidden in the shadows of X-ray projections (Figs 4.47 to 4.49).[1]

Temporomandibular Joint

Components of temporomandibular joint (TMJ), i.e. glenoid fossa, condylar head, sigmoid notch, subcondylar region, articular eminences of temporal bone are appreciated with limitation on conventional TMJ imaging techniques. Also superimposition of adjacent anatomical structure limits the diagnosis on these imaging techniques.

Cone beam computed tomography adequately shows the entire anatomy of TMJ components in various planes, i.e. sagittal, axial and coronal views. Osseous abnormalities involving the joint, trauma, pathology of TMJ are seen best on CBCT. Discal anatomy is observed best on magnetic resonance imaging (MRI) and ultrasound.

Coronal view demonstrates the medial and lateral pole of the condyle and its relation to glenoid fossa in frontal plane. Axial view also shows the medial and lateral pole of condyle in topographic view. Sagittal section reveals lateral aspect of condylar head with articular eminence. Bony changes are depicted clearly on CBCT images. Also 3D reconstruction allows visualization of structures from all directions, thus assisting in perfect diagnosis (Figs 4.50 to 4.53).

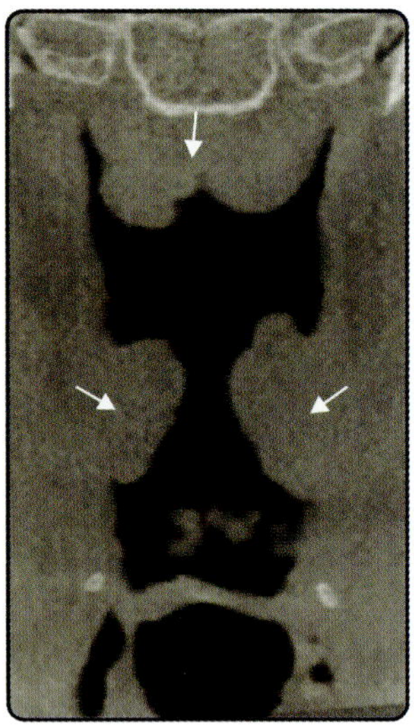

Figure 4.49: Coronal view showing airspace with enlarged adenoids

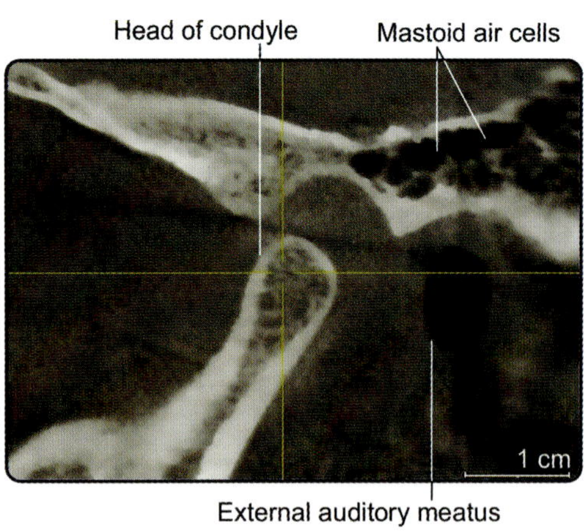

Figure 4.50: Sagittal view showing condylar head and external auditory meatus

An astute clinician will diagnose and treat the pathology only when they are being taught normal anatomical structures and its orientation on 3D imaging modality. This increases clinician's expertise and confidence in providing high-quality health care.

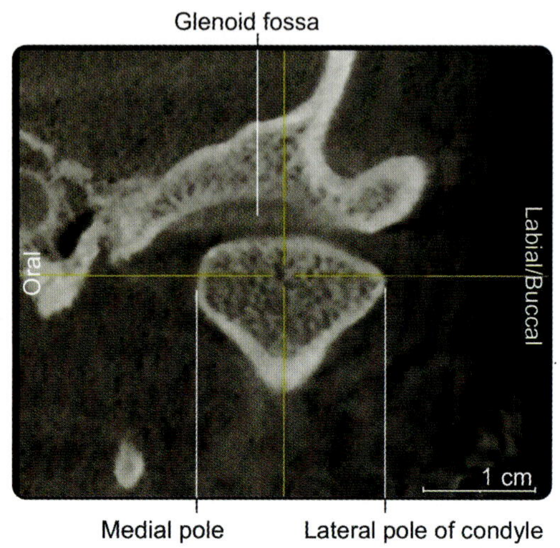

Figure 4.51: Coronal view showing both poles of condyle

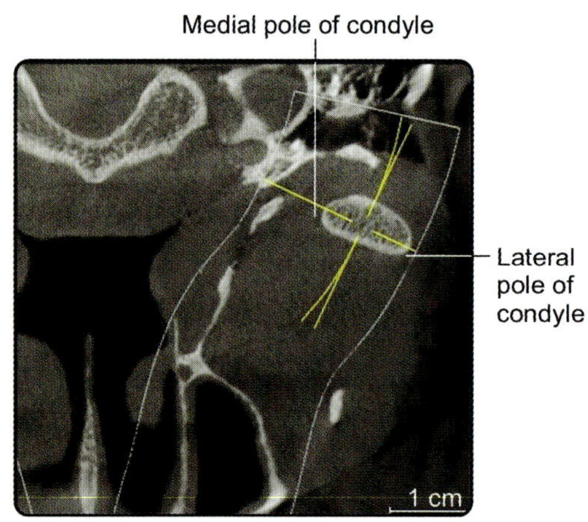

Figure 4.52: Axial view of temporomandibular joint (TMJ) showing both poles of condyles

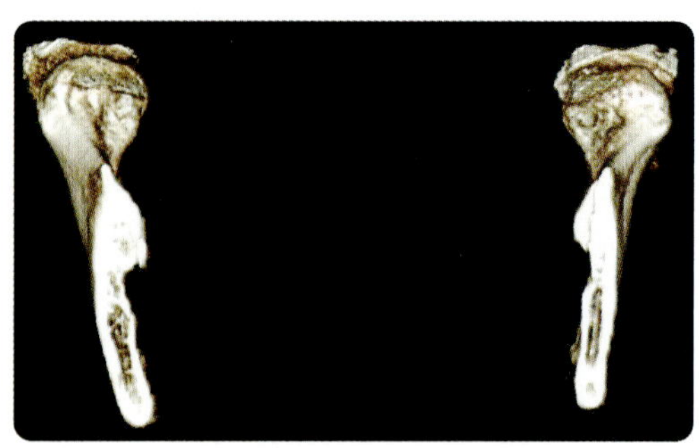

Figure 4.53: Three-dimensional reconstruction showing bilaterally condylar head

REFERENCES

1. Angelopoulos C. Cone beam tomographic imaging anatomy of the maxillofacial region. Dent Clin North Am. 2008;52(4):731-52.
2. Bornstein MM, Balsiger R, Sendi P, et al. Morphology of the nasopalatine canal and dental implant surgery: a radiographic analysis of 100 consecutive patients using limited cone-beam computed tomography. Clin Oral Implants Res. 2011;22(3):295-301.
3. Jaju PP, Jaju SP, Suvarna PV, et al. Dental CT: Third Eye in Dental Implants, 1st edition. New Delhi: Jaypee Brothers Medical Publishers (P) Ltd; 2013.
4. Lana JP, Carneiro PM, Machado Vde C, et al. Anatomic variations and lesions of the maxillary sinus detected in cone beam computed tomography for dental implants. Clin Oral Implants Res. 2012;23(12):1398-403.
5. Swirzinski KH, Edwards PC, Saini TS, et al. Length and geometric patterns of the greater palatine canal observed in cone beam computed tomography. International Journal of Dentistry. 2010;2010.
6. NS Norton. Netter's Head and Neck Anatomy for Dentistry. Philadelphia: Saunders; 2007.
7. Apostolakis D, Brown JE. The anterior loop of the inferior alveolar nerve: prevalence, measurement of its length and a recommendation for interforaminal implant installation based on cone beam CT imaging. Clin Oral Implants Res. 2012;23(9):1022-30.
8. Naitoh M, Hiraiwa Y, Aimiya H, et al. Accessory mental foramen assessment using cone-beam computed tomography. Oral Surg Oral Med Oral Pathol Oral Radiol Endod. 2009;107(2):289-94.

5 Chapter

Role of Cone Beam Computed Tomography in Prosthodontics

Prashant P Jaju, Sushma P Jaju

INTRODUCTION

Cone beam computed tomography (CBCT) plays an important role in the field of prosthetic dentistry. Replacement of missing teeth in the form of dental implants with designing of the future restoration via computer-aided design/computer-aided manufacturing (CAD/CAM) technology has revolutionized the prosthetic field. This chapter highlights the role of CBCT in prosthetic field, especially dental implants and CAD-CAM technology.

CONE BEAM COMPUTED TOMOGRAPHY IN DENTAL IMPLANTOLOGY

'Forewarned is forearmed,' is an old adage applied to the medical field and so is to the field of implant dentistry. Dental implants are gaining immense popularity and wide acceptance because they are the conservative method of replacing lost teeth and restore function with proprioception, esthetics and thereby revamp the self-esteem of the patients. The dental implant restorations have the highest survival rate compared with any other type of prosthesis to replace missing teeth. They do not decay or require endodontic treatment. They are also less prone to fracture and resist periodontal like disease better than teeth. Today, we see widespread clinical applications for implant procedures from the replacement of single teeth to extensive bone grafting for total reconstruction of maxillofacial skeleton needed as a result of tumor excision, trauma, etc. Implant dentistry has become an important tool for increasing the life expectancy of edentulous patients by improving the masticatory efficiency of the stomatognathic system. Patients with loss of teeth can be the victims of terrible social rejection, which includes loss of self-confidence and self-esteem, resulting from the overshadowing aspect of endpoint atrophy of the maxillofacial skeleton. CBCT has revolutionized the way dental implant practice is performed in dental clinics and hospitals. Past decades has shown a paradigm shift from a surgically driven to a prosthetically driven approach to dental implant therapy (Fig. 5.1). To improve the overall success of implant therapy with possible reduction in surgical and postoperative implant complications, implantologists should have three-dimensional (3D) information of bone volume and topography prior to implant placement.[1] Presurgical assessment of implant site by imaging techniques thereby allows accurate assessment of bone volume available, bone density, proximity to anatomical structures (Table 5.1).

Principles of Imaging for Dental Implant Assessment

The basic principles of radiology apply to imaging for implant evaluations. Images should have appropriate diagnostic quality and not contain artifacts that compromise anatomical structure assessments. Images should extend beyond the immediate area of interest to include areas that could be affected by implant placements. Practitioners should have appropriate training in operating radiographic

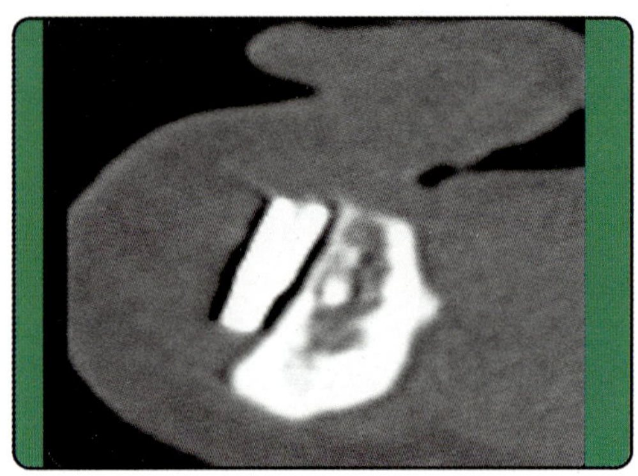

Figure 5.1: Lack of accurate assessment leads to improper positioning of implant

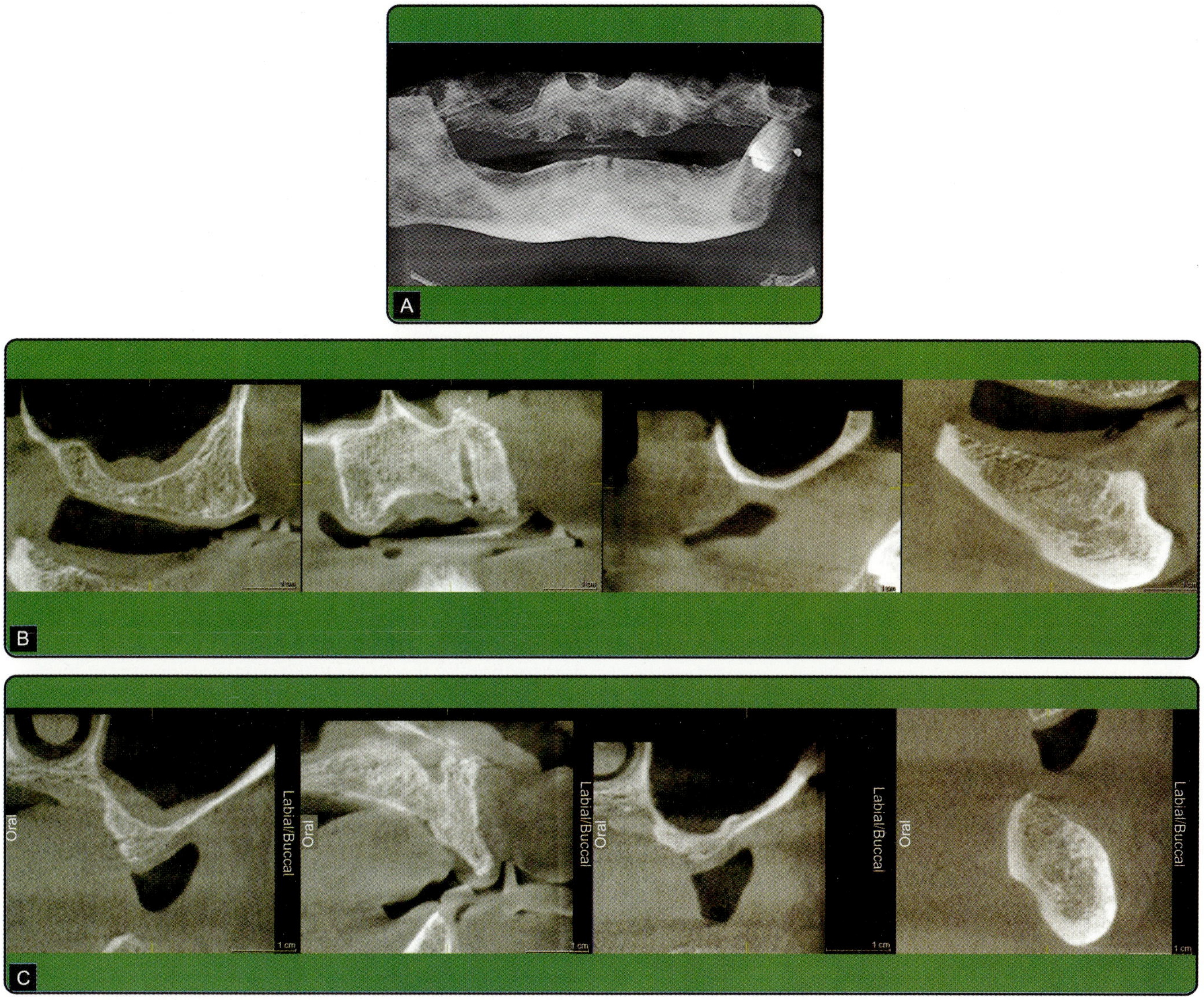

Figures 5.2A to C: Reconstructed panoramic image showing adequate bone volume. **A.** Reconstructed orthopantomograph (OPG); **B.** Tangential view; **C.** Cross-sectional view.

equipment and competence in interpreting images from the modality used. This training and competence should be maintained through continuing dental education courses. Such training should include a thorough review of normal maxillofacial anatomy, common anatomical variants and imaging signs of diseases and abnormalities. This is particularly important for computed tomography (CT) and CBCT imaging because of the complexity of structures within the expanded field of views (FOVs). The goal of radiographic selection criteria is to identify appropriate imaging modalities that complement the goals at each stage of implant therapy. The use of specific imaging is based on professional judgment (i.e. the clinician's professional opinion as to whether or not information from the clinical examination is inadequate and imaging is needed to formulate a diagnosis and a treatment plan, and/or for use at surgery) (Figs 5.2A to C).[2]

Cone beam computed tomography is the preferred option for implant dentistry, providing greater accuracy in measuring compared to 2D imaging, while utilizing lower doses of radiation.

Ridge Morphology

Buccolingual ridge pattern cannot be viewed on 2D radiographs, but CBCT provides with advantage of appreciating the type of alveolar ridge pattern present.[1]

Table 5.1: Comparison of imaging modalities in the field of dental implantology[2]

Imaging goal	Cephalometric	Periapical	*OPG	Tomography	CT†	CBCT‡
Bone height	1	3	2	3	4	4
Bone width	0	0	0	3	4	4
Long axis or ridge	0	0	0	3	4	4
Anatomy localization	1	1	1	3	4	4
Bone quality	0	2	2	2	4	3
Pathology identification	1	2	3	2	3	4
Jaw boundaries identification	1	0	2	3	4	4
Virtual planning	0	0	1	1	4	4
Guide fabrication	0	0	0	0	4	4
Communication aid	2	1	2	2	4	4
Benefit/Risk/Cost ratio	1	1	2	2	3	4

*OPG, occult pulmonary contusion; †CT, computed tomography; ‡CBCT, cone beam computed tomography.
Note: Ranking scores, 0 = no score, 1 = low value, 2 = mild value, 3 = moderate value, 4 = high value.

Cross-sectional images provide the implantologist the appearance of ridge patterns like irregular ridge, narrow crestal ridge and knife-shaped ridge. Also loss of cortical plates, undulating concavities can also be appreciated on cross-sectional images, which cannot be seen on panoramic image.[1] McGinvney et al and Schwartz et al concluded that three-dimensional images more accurately reflected the true osseous topography and considered it as a valuable diagnostic aid.[1] In case of compromised jaw bone in terms of quality and/or quantity of bone, panoramic technique is an inefficient imaging tool. This dictates additional imaging in 2D/3D, especially when there is risks and doubts about treatment outcome, 3D imaging may prove indispensable (Figs 5.3A and B).[2]

Quantity of Available Bone at Implant Site

Available bone is the amount of bone in the edentulous area considered for osseointegration of the implant. As a general guideline a distance of 1.5 mm is maintained for surgical error between the implant and any adjacent landmark. The chances of successful implantation are increased by more bone being available for anchorage and distribution of masticatory forces. Cortical bone is best suited to provide support for implants. Accurate estimates of the alveolar bone height and width are mandatory for selecting the appropriate implant size and determining the degree of angulation of the edentulous alveolar ridge. The assessment of the angulation of the alveolar ridge provides information regarding the proper insertion path of the fixture. The angulation of the alveolar bone represents the root trajectory in relation to the occlusal plane. Measurement of the height and width at the proposed implant site can be done on the films itself as 'life size' or it can determined by the PC of the implantologist.

Maxilla

For maxillary anterior region, the height of the available ridge can be calculated from the crest of ridge to inferior border of nasal fossa. For maxillary posterior region, the height of the ridge can be calculated from the superior border of crest of ridge to the inferior border of maxillary sinus. For mandibular anterior region, the height of the ridge can be calculated from the crest of ridge to inferior border of mandible. For mandibular posterior region, the height of the ridge can be calculated from

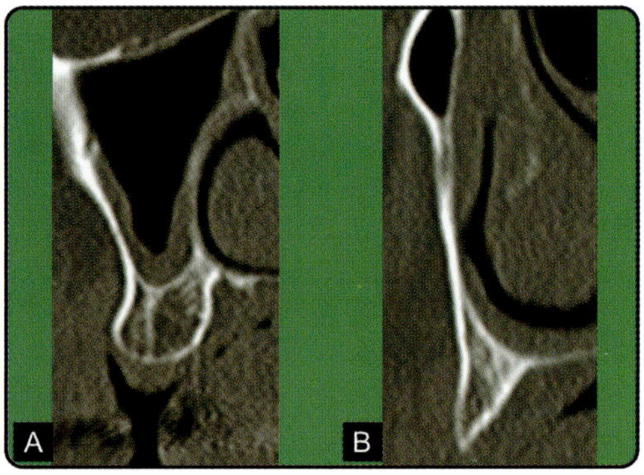

Figures 5.3A and B: Types of ridges. **A.** Rectangular shaped; **B.** Triangular shaped.

the crest of ridge to superior border of inferior alveolar canal (Fig. 5.4).

Authors have observed that many radiologists provide the width by measuring from the outer cortical plates. There would be instances where a knife-shaped ridge may be present or where insufficient width would be present, until the implantologist perform osteotomy to achieve adequate width. CBCT helps us to determine the amount of bone required to be removed during the osteotomy procedure for adequate acquisition of buccolingual width. This function can be performed by utilizing the linear scale tool present on the software. An interesting clinically relevant classification can be used for determining the available bone as suggested by Chanavaz and Donazzan. This classification is termed as Chanavaz and Donazzan French Volumetric Classification (1986) (Table 5.2).[1]

This classification gives a clear idea about the type of bone available at the implant sites. Presence of type A bone will be difficult to obtain, if the patient do not report very early for implant. Generally, the implantologist are encountered with type B bone in their clinical practice. Amount of bone loss occurring at the 1st year after the tooth loss is 10 times greater than the following years. There are greater chances of type A bone in maxillary posterior region as maxillary teeth are generally not lost at an early age as compared with mandibular first molar, which tend to be affected by caries very early. Also it has been reported that atrophy of the maxillary arch proceeds at a slower rate than in the mandible. The posterior mandible resorbs approximately four times faster than the anterior mandible. The original height of available bone in the mandible is twice that of maxilla. The changes in anterior maxilla ridge dimension can be very dramatic both in height and width up to 70% especially when multiple extractions are performed. The residual ridge shifts palatally in the maxillary and lingually in the mandible as related to tooth position at the expense of buccal cortical plate in all areas of jaw. Literature states that the decrease in bone begins in fourth decade and is linear.[1]

Table 5.2: Chanavaz and Donazzan French volumetric classification (1986)

Category	Dimensions	Other features
A	Height: 9 mm Width: 5 mm	Abundant bone in all dimensions with intact basal bone
B	Height: 9 mm Width: 3 mm	Abundant bone except width, intact basal bone, partially resorbed alveolar bone (after 5–9 year of extraction)
C	Inadequate bone	Totally resorbed alveolar bone, intact basal bone
D	Severe bone atrophy	Totally resorbed alveolar bone, partially resorbed basal bone except symphysis region and external oblique ridge

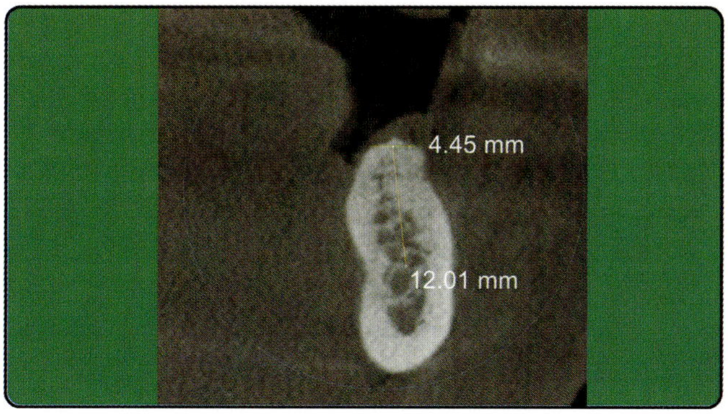

Figure 5.4: Measurement of available bone at proposed implant site

After the measurement at the proposed implant site, current CBCT softwares allow virtual placement of implants allowing the implantologist to know the precise location, angulation of the implants. Implant library available in the CBCT software allows placing of the virtual implant of the choice of the implantologist thereby reducing the armamentarium at surgery stage (Figs 5.5A to E and 5.6).

Generic or customized abutment and sleeve selection is also possible, thus allowing prospective prosthetic component to be visualized on the computer screen and improving the overall success rate (Figs 5.7 and 5.8A and B).

Height or Width of Implant

Which is the Critical Parameter?

The width of implant decreases the stress by increasing the surface area. This may also reduce the length requirement. For every 0.5 mm increase in width there is an increased surface area between 10% and 15%. Since the greatest stresses are concentrated at the crestal region of implant, width is more significant than the length for an implant design. In patients with triangular-shaped cross section, osteoplasty should be advised to obtain greater width of bone, although of reduced height. This rule was not applied in anterior maxilla as most edentulous ridges exhibited a labial concavity in the incisor area resulting an hour glass configuration.[1]

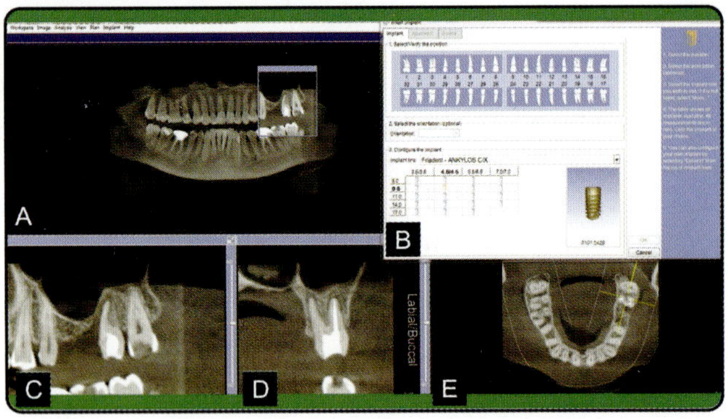

Figures 5.5A to E: Virtual implant placement from Galileo (Sirona) implant library. **A.** Reconstructed orthopantomograph (OPG); **B.** Implant library; **C.** Tangential view; **D.** Cross-sectional view; **E.** Axial view.

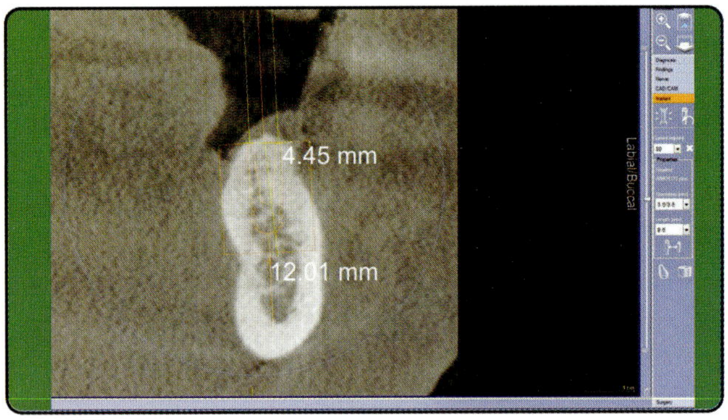

Figure 5.6: Virtual implant placement at implant site from Galileo (Sirona)

Does Sex Affect the Quantity of Bone?

Female patients have a tendency for greater bone resorption. Following rapid initial resorption, the rate decreases and then continues at about 0.1 mm per year in male and about 0.4 mm per year in female. This can be attributed to the decreased estrogen level in female patients. Females are more prone to osteoporosis and subsequently there is faster resorption of bone. The age-associated bone loss is about 1% in women and 0.5% in males annually. Women represent a greater percentage of patients with residual ridge resorption than men.[1]

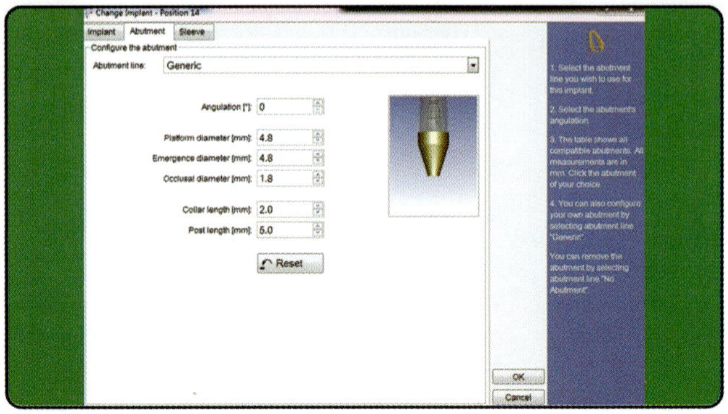

Figure 5.7: Abutment and sleeve selection from Galileo (Sirona)

Quality of Bone at Implant Sites

The term bone quality is commonly used in implant treatment and in reports on implant success and failure. Lindh et al emphasized that bone density, bone mineral density (BMD) and bone quality are not synonymous.[3] Bone quality encompasses factors other than bone density such as skeletal size, the architecture and 3D orientation of the trabecular and matrix properties. Bone quality is not only a matter of mineral content but also of structure. It has been shown that the quality and quantity of bone available at the implant site are very important local patient factors in determining the success of dental implants.[4] Bone quality is categorized into four groups—groups 1–4 or type I–IV bone quality index (BQI).[5]

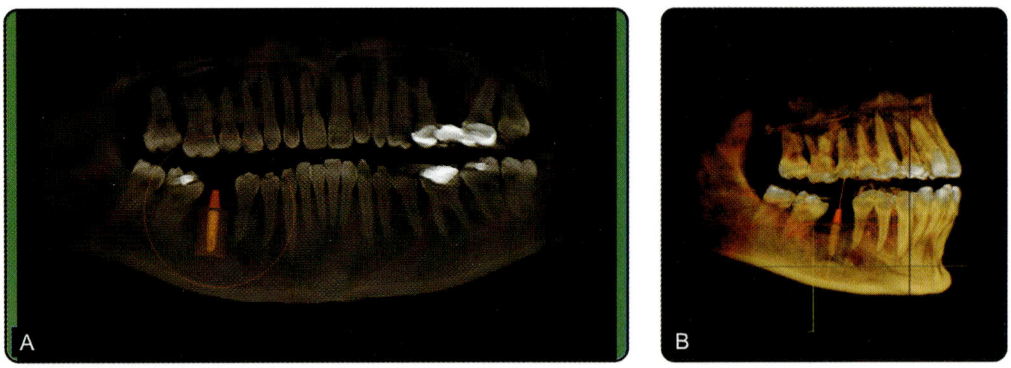

Figures 5.8A and B: Reconstructed panoramic and three-dimensional reconstruction showing virtual implant placement. **A.** Reconstructed orthopantomograph; **B.** Three-dimensional reconstruction.

- Type I: Homogeneous cortical bone
- Type II: Thick cortical bone with marrow cavity
- Type III: Thin cortical bone with dense trabecular bone of good strength
- Type IV: Very thin cortical bone with low density trabecular bone of poor strength.

In the jaws, an implant placed in poor-quality bone with thin cortex and low-density trabeculae (type IV bone) has a higher chance of failure compared with the other types of bones. This low-density bone is often found in the posterior maxilla and several studies report higher implant failure rates in this region.

Bone density can be obtained from CT units and expressed in the form of Hounsfield units (HU). The HU is not part of the SI system. In fact it is a practical unit that represents the relative deviation of the measured linear attenuation of a material from that of water X-ray beams used for diagnostic radiology are not monochromatic and hence composed of photons with a broad spectrum of energies. This is the fundamental reason why HU value for a tissue obtained from one CT system may not be the same as that obtained with a different CT system or even with the same machine if different technique factors are used.[6]

Unlike CT units, current CBCT units do not use a standard scaling system. Methods have been proposed to convert CT numbers measured on CBCT scans to HU. However, such methods make the implicit assumption that the relationship between CT numbers and X-ray attenuation is uniform through the CBCT image volume. Several factors like beam hardening, artifacts from metallic restorations and scattered radiation contribute to the inhomogeneity of CT numbers on CBCT scans. It has been reported that even same anatomic region on CBCT scans may not demonstrate same CT numbers. In general, smaller irradiated and reconstructed volumes (small FOVs) are less prone to inaccurate CT numbers caused by scattered radiation and by non-ideal geometry; therefore whenever there is no need for large volume coverage, a small FOV should be used instead of a large FOV.[6]

Gray-level values from CBCT images are influenced by device and scanning settings. For HUs on CBCT to be used with confidence, the accuracy of the HU should be known, so that the clinician can assess whether or not the HUs can be used for specific clinical tasks.[6] With more advanced CBCT software methods, it should be possible to improve the accuracy of CBCT HU values for determining bone densities at implant sites. Thus, it can be concluded that CBCT provides a subjective assessment of bone quality and not objective assessment.

Professional judgment varies depending on the skill, competence, knowledge and experience of the clinician. Specific considerations must include clinical and anatomical complexity, potential risks of complications and esthetic outcomes. The following selection criteria recommendations provide literature based, consensus derived and clinical guidance for practitioners on the appropriate imaging (with particular relevance to CBCT) at each phase of dental-implant therapy.

Recommendations by AAOMR for Role of CBCT in Dental Implantology[7]

Recommendation 1: Panoramic radiography should be used as the imaging modality of choice in the initial evaluation of the dental implant patient.

Recommendation 2: Use intraoral periapical radiography to supplement the preliminary information from panoramic radiography.

Recommendation 3: Do not use cross-sectional imaging including CBCT as an initial diagnostic imaging examination.

Recommendation 4: The radiographic examination of any potential implant site should include cross-sectional imaging orthogonal to the site of interest.

Recommendation 5: CBCT should be considered as the imaging modality of choice for preoperative cross-sectional imaging of potential implant sites.

Recommendation 6: CBCT should be considered when clinical conditions indicate a need for augmentation procedures or site development before placement of dental implants:

- Sinus augmentation
- Block or particulate bone grafting
- Ramus or symphysis grafting
- Assessment of impacted teeth in the field of interest
- Evaluation of prior traumatic injury.

Recommendation 7: CBCT imaging should be considered if bone reconstruction and augmentation procedures (e.g. ridge preservation or bone grafting) have been performed to treat bone volume deficiencies before implant placement.

Recommendation 8: In the absence of clinical signs or symptoms, use intraoral periapical radiography for the postoperative assessment of implants. Panoramic radiographs may be indicated for more extensive implant therapy cases.

Recommendation 9: Use cross-sectional imaging (particularly CBCT) immediately postoperatively only if the patient presents with implant mobility or altered sensation, especially if the fixture is in the posterior mandible.

Recommendation 10: Do not use CBCT imaging for periodic review of clinically asymptomatic implants.

Recommendation 11: Cross-sectional imaging, optimally CBCT, should be considered if implant retrieval is anticipated.

CBCT-GUIDED IMPLANT SURGERY

Type and size of the planned implants, its position within the bone, its relationship to the planned restoration and adjacent teeth and/or implants, and its proximity to vital structures can be determined before performing surgery. This is possible with integration of CBCT scans with CAD/CAM technology (e.g. CEREC, Sirona Germany). Computer-generated surgical guides can be fabricated from the virtual treatment plan. These surgical guides are used by the implantologist to place the planned implants in the patient's mouth in the same position as in the virtual treatment plan, allowing more accurate and predictable implant placement and reduced patient morbidity.[8] Surgical guides are not indicated for every case. Indications are as follows:

- Three or more implants in a row
- Proximity to vital anatomic structures
- Problems related to the proximity of adjacent teeth
- Questionable bone volume
- Implant position that is critical to the planned restoration
- Flapless implant placement
- Multiple unit or full arch immediate restorations with or without extractions and immediate placement.

Conventional surgical stents to aid in implant positioning have been used in implant dentistry for many years. Guides are fabricated from vacuform shells with the buccal or palatal/lingual facings of the planned restorations or more complex with 2 mm drill holes or metal tubes. There is a lack of correlation in these appliances between the planned restoration and the underlying bony anatomy. With the use of computer-guided implant surgical guides this anatomic relationship can be predictably established and considered before surgery.[8] Gutta-percha, barium sulfate and lead foils have been traditionally used for fabrication of surgical guides. Bone and soft tissue loss from periodontal disease and atrophy, long-term denture wear and sinus pneumatization can make it difficult to predictably use a traditional surgical-guides (Figs 5.9A to C).[8]

Three types of computer-generated surgical guides are currently available:

1. Tooth supported.
2. Mucosa supported.
3. Bone supported.

Tooth supported guides are used in partially edentulous cases. This surgical guide is designed to rest on other teeth in the arch for accuracy of guide fit. Mucosal supported guides are used primarily in fully edentulous cases and are designed to rest on the mucosa. Accurate interarch bite registrations are the utmost importance when using these guides to assure accurate surgical guide positioning and placement of securing screws/pins before placement of implants. Bone supported guides can be used in partially or fully edentulous cases, but are used primarily in fully edentulous cases in which significant ridge atrophy is present and good seating of a mucosa supported guides is questionable. Currently only SimPlant (Materialize) manufactures bone supporting surgical guides.[8]

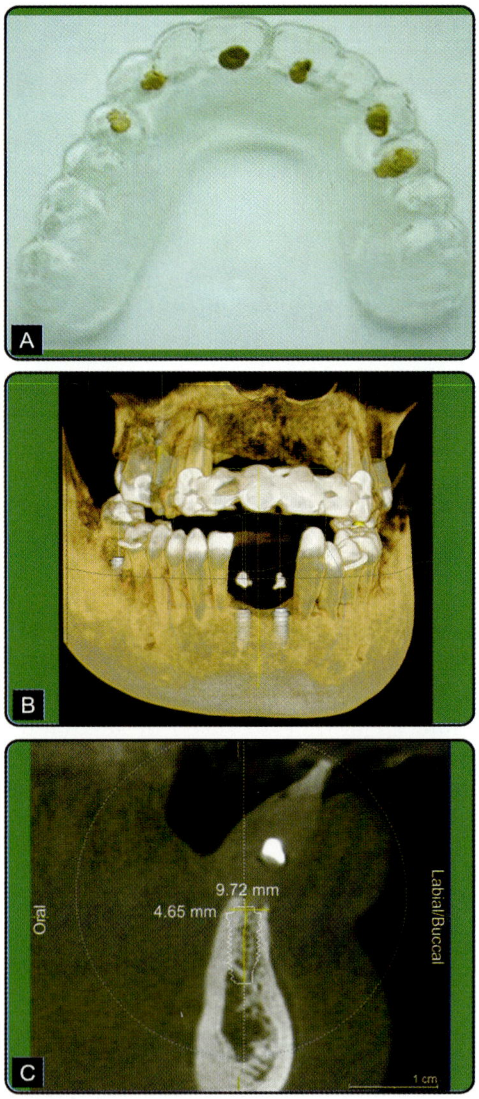

Figures 5.9A to C: Conventional radiographic guide using gutta-percha. **A.** Acrylic radiographic guide; **B.** Three-dimensional reconstruction; **C.** Cross-sectional view.

Integration of Cone Beam Computed Tomography and CAD/CAM[9]

Dental CAD/CAM technology is used in both dental laboratories and dental offices for multiple restorative applications. Chairside CAD/CAM systems for dental offices offer dentists the opportunity to design, mill and place ceramic restorations in a single appointment. As implants become the treatment of choice for fixed tooth replacement, dentists also are considering using chairside CAD/CAM systems as a restorative solution for implant prosthetics. A predictable CAD/CAM technique for dental implantology could satisfy patients' preference for convenience and dentists' desire for predictable, long-term restorations. Clinical research provides documentation of the success of ceramic restorations created using the Chairside Economical Restoration of Esthetic Ceramics (CEREC) system (Sirona Dental Systems, Charlotte, North Carolina).[9] As the technology has evolved, it also has been used to restore dental implants.

The primary emphasis in a surgery-focused approach to implant placement is on the anatomy, bone physiology and surgical success. The restorative demands of the case may be secondary when determining the placement of the implant fixture. During the restorative phase, compensation for deviations in implant fixture location involves the use of complex custom prosthetics components. A technique that requires custom prosthetics designed after surgical placement of the endosseous dental implant does not allow for the implant to be restored in a single visit because of the required laboratory fabrication process. Dentists need to consider the restorative goal and surgical requirements to plan optimally for the surgical placement of implants. This process requires a plan for the final restoration's optimal function, esthetics and biomechanics before making the surgical plan. The traditional technique for such planning begins with using diagnostic casts, impressions and clinical records. Using the diagnostic casts, the dentist or laboratory technician produces a wax-up to simulate the desired restorative outcome. A stone duplication of the wax-up is necessary for processing either a laboratory surgical guide to help with traditional implant placement or a radiographic scanning appliance for subsequent diagnostic implant planning. This workflow involves multiple patient appointments and separate laboratory procedures involving the clinician and the laboratory technician before the implant can be placed. Because of procedural complexity, the clinician may favor a surgically focused technique for implant placement and treat the restorative process as secondary.[9]

Sirona Dental Systems introduced a combination of 3D radiographic imaging and 3D planning by integrating CEREC Acquisition Center (AC) design with Galileos (Sirona Dental Systems) cone beam computed tomographic (CBCT) imaging to facilitate comprehensive implant treatment. Galileos CEREC integration (GCI) simplifies restorative-focused implant placements through the use of intraoral surface data (the digital impression) and radiographic data. The GCI technique gives dentists the opportunity to plan optimum prosthetic and surgical outcomes for implants during the diagnostic and planning phases of treatment, while minimizing the number of procedures and increasing workflow efficiency.[9]

By using GCI software, the clinician can identify the restorative requirements virtually including proper restorative material thickness around the long axis of the planned implant, depth of restorative interface and emergence profile. Such information may help the dentist decide whether to use stock abutments or custom anatomic abutments. Until now, the convenience of chairside CAD/CAM for implant restoration was limited by material strength. The ability to plan implant placement with restorative vision by using the GCI software combined with a restorative material whose properties are an improvement over those of conventional glass ceramics provides the dentist with a viable comprehensive protocol for implant placement and chairside CAD/CAM all ceramic restorative success.[9]

Clinical Workflows

There are a number of possible workflows that can be followed when using the GCI technique.[9]

Single-implant workflow

For a single implant site, the clinical workflow begins with obtaining a digital impression by using CEREC AC and Galileos CBCT during the initial consultation. Instead of using conventional impressions and diagnostic wax-ups, the dentist can use the digital impression to record the surface anatomy and design an ideal restoration virtually. The digital impression is obtained by coating the tooth and gingival surfaces lightly with an optical reflective medium to create a uniform surface and by using the CEREC AC Bluecam to acquire image data. Obtaining the digital impression includes capturing both the edentulous quadrant and the opposing quadrant in separate image catalogs. The virtual models created from the digital impression are articulated by using an additional image recorded when the patient is in maximum intercuspation (buccal bite technique).

The dentist or technician uses CEREC biogeneric software (version 3.80, Sirona Dental Systems) to create virtual wax-ups of planned restorations that include parameters such as occlusal contacts, proximal contacts, emergence profile, proximal contours and the desired material thickness for optimal strength of the ceramic restoration.

In addition to the optical impression, a Galileos CBCT scan of the patient is obtained by means of a stock scanning bite plate (SICAT, Bonn, Germany). The bite plate is seated clinically by using the bite registration material. The bite plate is converted to the surgical guide at a later stage. The Galileos CBCT scans provide a 3D volume image of the hard tissue that can be evaluated by using software to evaluate radiographic sections of the anatomy that correlate one-to-one without distortion or magnification.[9]

The CAD/CAM and CBCT systems provide comprehensive diagnostic data. The acquisition of surface anatomy and radiographic anatomy data allows the dentist to design and plan treatment, and order precision surgical guides for guided implant placement in one visit. The process requires the dentist to combine the data sets from the two systems by using GCI software that uses sophisticated algorithms to match common data points. The dentist need only to identify common features between the two digital images (for example, placing an identification marker on tooth number two in the CEREC AC image and on tooth number two in the Galileos image) to allow the software to correlate the data. Once combined, the CEREC AC data are visible within the Galileos software, allowing the dentist to plan the implant position as it relates to both the prosthetic and surgical requirements of the case.[9] Within the software, a library of implant systems from which to plan implant positioning relative to restorative and surgical goals is available. Once the dentist determines the type of implant and surgical positioning, he/she can order the surgical guide. The patient's data set and scanning template are sent to SICAT for fabrication of the implant surgical guide. The surgical guides are compatible with most of the available implant systems. This workflow allows for guided surgical implantation during the patient's second visit. Implant placement accuracy when using the SICAT surgical guides is within 500 micrometers of planned implant placement location.[9]

Once osseointegration is complete, the restorative phase of treatment can begin and the dentist can use the data from CEREC AC and Galileos that were used during the planning phase to understand the restorative options in advance. The dentist can seat a stock or standard abutment clinically and scan it intraorally with CEREC AC to fabricate a full-contour restoration similar to a preparation for a crown on a natural tooth.[9]

After the dentist seats the abutment clinically, he/she can fill the screw access hole with a retrievable material to protect the screw for future access. Tissue retraction is necessary to visualize the abutment margin. The dentist can retract the gingivae by using conventional means such as a retraction cord, retraction gels and pastes and laser treatment. Once the dentist has isolated the abutment, he/she follows the conventional chairside optical impression protocol by using CEREC AC Bluecam. Within the CEREC AC software, the dentist can evaluate and confirm the abutment's restorative margin, interproximal contacts, occlusal contacts, emergence profile and soft-tissue support. Essentially, the dentist can design a final crown by using the CEREC AC software and customize it to fit the restorative environment, chairside. The dentist selects IPS e.max CAD and sends the data to the inLab MC XL (Sirona Dental Systems) milling chamber for chairside CAM of the crown. After the dentist retrieves the restoration from the milling chamber, he/she can evaluate the restoration clinically and adjust it if necessary, while it is in the precrystallized state. The dentist can introduce custom staining and glazing before the restoration is crystallized to final lithium disilicate transformation for optimal strength and esthetics.[9]

Custom abutment and crown workflow

Another workflow relies on the dentist's sending the CEREC AC digital impression data to a dental laboratory by using the CEREC connect software (Sirona Dental Systems) via the CEREC inLab conflict of interest: None (Sirona Dental Systems) system to fabricate a custom abutment and crown.[9]

CONCLUSION

Cone beam computed tomography, CAD/CAM integration is the future of prosthetic and implant field and it is the way forward.

REFERENCES

1. Jaju PP. Suvarna PV. Dental CT third Eye in dental implants. In: Jaju PP, Jaju SP, Suvarna PV, Dedhia P (Eds). Dental CT in Implantology, 1st edition. New Delhi, India: Jaypee Brothers Medical Publishers (P) Ltd; 2013.
2. Worthington P, Rubenstein J, Hatcher DC. The role of cone-beam computed tomography in the planning and placement of implants. J Am Dent Assoc. 2010;141 Suppl 3:19S-24S.
3. Lindh C, Obrant K, Petersson A. Maxillary bone mineral density and its relationship to the bone mineral density of the lumbar spine and hip. Oral Surg Oral Med Oral Pathol Oral Radiol Endod. 2004;98(1):102-9.

4. Drage NA, Palmer RM, Blake G, et al. A comparison of bone mineral density in the spine, hip and jaws of edentulous subjects. Clin Oral Implants Res. 2007;18(4):496-500.
5. Lekholm U, Zarb GA. Patient selection and preparation. In: Brånemark PI, Zarb GA, Albrektsson T (Eds). Tissue Integrated Prostheses: Osseointegration in Clinical Dentistry, 1st edition. Chicago: Quintessence Publishing; 1985. pp. 199-209.
6. Molteni R. Prospects and challenges of rendering tissue density in Hounsfield units for cone beam computed tomography. Oral Surg Oral Med Oral Pathol Oral Radiol. 2013;116(1):105-19.
7. Tyndall DA, Price JB, Tetradis S, et al. Position statement of the American Academy of Oral and Maxillofacial Radiology on selection criteria for the use of radiology in dental implantology with emphasis on cone beam computed tomography. Oral Surg Oral Med Oral Pathol Oral Radiol. 2012;113(6):817-26.
8. Orentlicher G, Abboud M. Guided surgery for implant therapy. Dent Clin North Am. 2011;55(4):715-44.
9. Patel N. Integrating three-dimensional digital technologies for comprehensive implant dentistry. J Am Dent Assoc. 2010;141(2):20S-4S.

6

Chapter

Role of Cone Beam Computed Tomography in Orthodontics and Airway Analysis

Avani Dixit Gandhi

INTRODUCTION

Malocclusions and craniofacial anomalies adversely affect quality of life. Orthodontics and dentofacial orthopedic treatment addresses the correction of malocclusions and facial disproportions due to dental/skeletal discrepancies to provide esthetic, psychosocial and functional improvements.

The five major functional components of the face are:

1. Cranium and cranial base.
2. Skeletal maxilla.
3. Skeletal mandible.
4. Maxillary dentition and alveolar process.
5. Mandibular dentition and alveolar process.

The golden standard for orthodontic records is the attempt to achieve an accurate reproduction of the real anatomical structures or the 'anatomic truth'.

The purpose of radiographic imaging in orthodontics is to supplement or support clinical diagnosis in the pretreatment assessment of the orthodontic patient. Imaging may also be performed during treatment to assess the effects of therapy and post-treatment to monitor the outcome. Imaging for a specific orthodontic patient occurs in at least three stages:

1. Selection of the most appropriate radiographic imaging technique.
2. Acquisition of appropriate images.
3. Interpretation of the images obtained, sometimes followed by a repeat of these steps.

Since past many years, two-dimensional (2D) imaging modalities have been utilized for diagnosing and treatment planning to achieve movement in three-dimensional (3D) space. Although, orthopantomographs, periapical radiographs and cephalograms although extremely useful in orthodontic planning, and analyzing skeletal and dental relationships, leaves some unanswered questions owing to their 2D scope. Lateral and posteroanterior cephalograms were introduced to orthodontics in the early 1930s by Broadbent in United States of America and Hofrath in Germany. They obtained these radiographs using cephalostats to facilitate reproducible head positioning for films taken at different time points.[1] A lateral cephalogram is one of the orthodontic records that provide information about the sagittal and vertical relations of:

- Craniofacial skeleton
- Soft tissue profile
- Dentition
- Pharynx
- Cervical vertebrae.

Image magnification and distortion are the part of 2D radiography. With lateral cephalograms, structures on the left side are magnified less than the same structures on the right because of proximity to the film. With panoramic imaging, the amounts of horizontal and vertical magnification vary as objects may be placed outside the focal trough. Steiner wrote in 1953 about the use of cephalogram films "It has been claimed by many that it is a tool of the research laboratory and that the difficulties and expense of its use in clinical practice are not justified."[2] The cephalometric landmarks can only be identified in 2D radiographs by a sound knowledge of the anatomy of skull and also the radiographic appearance of each structure, and the criteria for identification of each anatomical cephalometric point.

CONE BEAM COMPUTED TOMOGRAPHY IN ORTHODONTICS

With the introduction of 3D radiography, these errors were minimized. Modern cone beam computer tomography (CBCT) systems applied to oral and maxillofacial regions provide a helpful diagnostic tool in orthodontics. This technology eliminated the errors of the conventional radiographs (magnification, image distortion, superimposition of anatomical structures) and the drawbacks that medical computed tomography (CT) presented like high -economic costs, high-radiation doses. CBCT offers the distinct advantage of 1:1 geometry, which allows accurate measurements of objects and dimensions.

Applications of Cone Beam Computed Tomography in Orthodontics[3]

Localization of Ectopic, Impacted and Supernumerary Teeth

The prevalence of impacted maxillary canines is approximately 0.9%–3.0%.[4,5] The ratio of palatal to labial impactions has been shown to be as high as 9:1.[6] In the past, orthodontists have used the tube shift technique to compare two periapical radiographs taken at different beam angles to determine the facial/lingual position of the impacted canine. This same lingual, opposite buccal rule is helpful in determining whether the impacted canine is labial or lingual to the incisor roots. However, the extent of displacement is difficult to determine. The CBCT imaging is precise in determining the labial/lingual and also the exact angulation of the impacted canine. These 3D images aid in determining the proximity of adjacent incisor and premolar roots, which helps in determining the vector of force that should be used to move the tooth into the arch with a lesser chance of adjacent root resorption.[3] Maxillary central incisors can be impacted and displaced subsequent to the presence of a mesiodens. The position of these teeth and the crown root morphology can be evaluated. This knowledge can help determine the need of retaining and placing traction on these impacted teeth. 2D radiographs, especially panoramic ones, can make definitive diagnosis difficulties. The CBCT image allows a more accurate view to help determine the presence and position of these teeth (Figs 6.1A to D and 6.2A to C).[3]

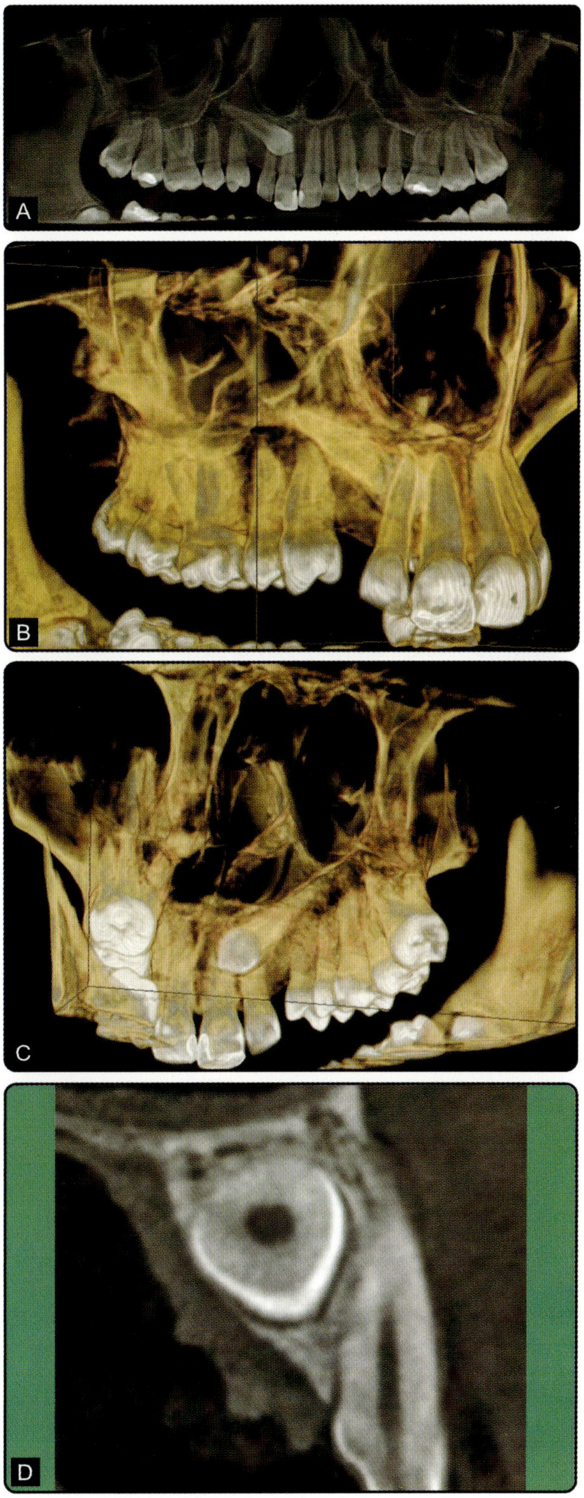

Figures 6.1A to D: Impacted right canine. **A.** Panoramic radiograph showing impacted right canine; **B.** Three-dimensional buccal view showing mesiodistally impacted right canine; **C.** Three-dimensional palatal view showing mesiodistally impacted right canine; **D.** Cross-sectional view showing relationship of impacted canine and central incisor.

Assessment of Root Resorption, Both from Ectopically Erupting Teeth as Result of Orthodontic Treatment Side Effect

Most root resorption involved in orthodontic treatment can be readily viewed on periapical radiographs. However, resorption that occurs on the facial or lingual side of the tooth is difficult to ascertain and quantify with this 2D view. CBCT scanning allows for better viewing of resorption on either of these surfaces.[7] However, the most important relationship of CBCT imaging to root resorption may

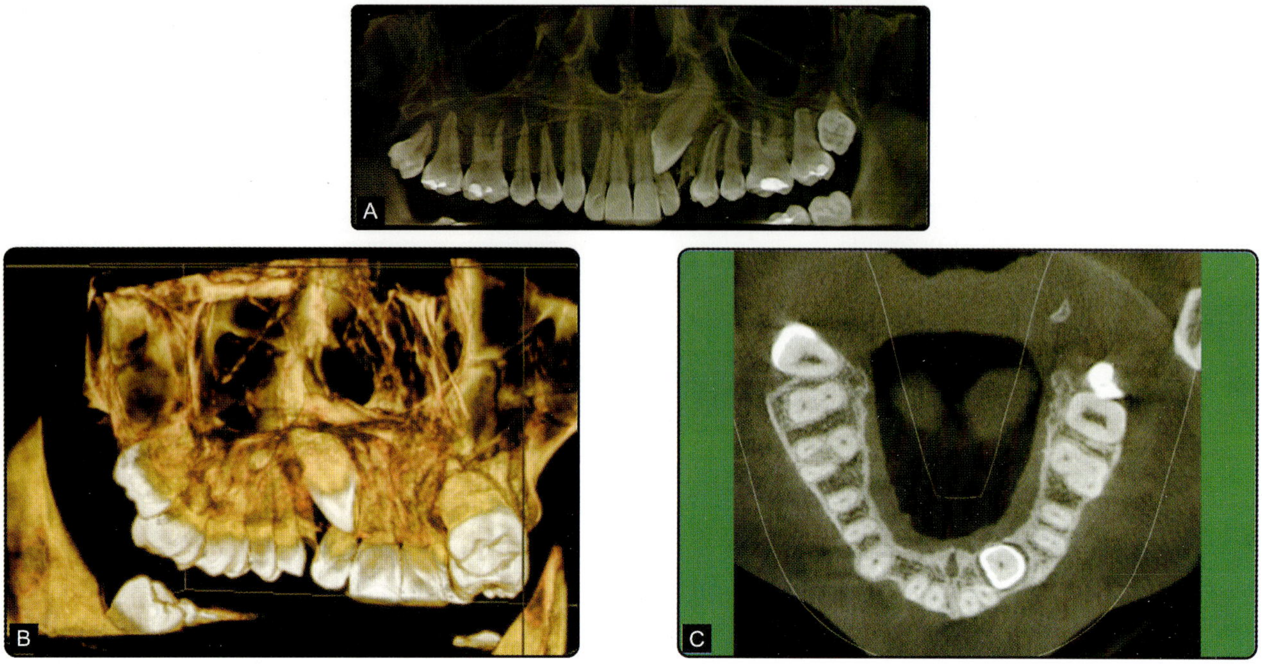

Figures 6.2A to C: Impacted canine. **A.** Impacted canine on left side with over-retained deciduous canine seen on panoramic; **B.** Three-dimensional view; **C.** Axial view.

be that of determining maxillary canine eruption position and its possible relationship with future spontaneous resorption of the adjacent lateral and central incisors. Removal of the deciduous canine adjacent to the impacted permanent canine has been shown to be effective, if accomplished early.[8]

Bony Dimensions in All Three Planes of Space

Using CBCT scans, alveolar bone can be assessed from all aspects not only on the mesial and distal surfaces of the tooth. This allows for the assessment of the width of available bone for buccolingual movement of teeth during orthodontic management especially in cases requiring arch expansion or labial movement of incisors. Fenestrations, dehiscence and/or external apical root resorption can be precisely visualized on the 3D images. Evaluation of alveolar bone volume, which is especially important in periodontal compromised adult orthodontic patients, is one of the beneficial uses of CBCT in orthodontics.[9]

Asymmetry Evaluation

Asymmetry evaluation can be difficult to evaluate the bony asymmetry of orthodontic patients using cephalometric and panoramic radiographs. Superimposition of structures, patient positioning, and distortion makes it difficult and unreliable. For instance, the comparison of the condyle and ramus lengths can be important to the occlusion of an orthodontic patient. Direct measurements of these structures can be made with CBCT imaging by comparing the right and left sides. Evaluation of mandibular asymmetry by the way of CBCT imaging eliminates positioning problems. Imaging can provide measurements of mandibular anatomy either through 2D panoramic reconstructions or the entire 3D data package.[10]

The unilateral nature of posterior crossbites can be diagnosed more specifically. The determination as to the presence of a truly unilateral crossbite versus one subsequent to a shift of the mandible into centric occlusion can be enhanced. A determination of an asymmetric maxilla or mandible can be accomplished more easily by viewing and measuring the bones in 3D. The orthodontist can view these structures in various angulations using the data taken in only one scan instead of using numerous 2D radiographic views.[3]

Cleft Lip and Palate

Estimation of the size (dimensions) of the osseous defects and the spatial relationship of the defect to other important anatomic structures are difficult to obtain in 2D images. CBCT can provide the cleft's exact anatomic relationships and bone thickness around the existing teeth in proximity to the cleft or clefts (Figs 6.3A to E). This information is invaluable for the grafting procedures planned and for possible tooth movement in the existing dentition.[3]

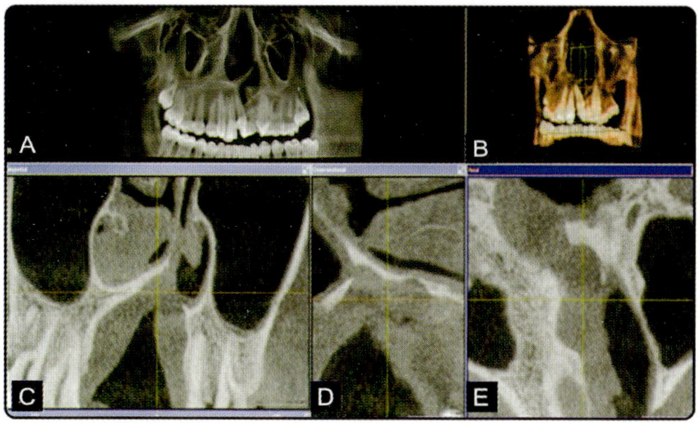

Figures 6.3A to E: Extend of cleft defect clearly seen on cone beam computed tomography (CBCT) imaging; **A.** Orthopantomogram showing the cleft defect; **B.** Three-dimensional reconstruction showing extend of cleft defect; **C.** Sagittal view; **D.** Cross sectional view; **E.** Axial view.

Airway

Using lateral cephalometric radiographs, the orthodontist may evaluate the airway in a 2D manner. Many studies have been accomplished and various analyses established in this way.[9-13] All this evaluation, however, is limited by the fact that we are looking at a flat projection seen in a sagittal or coronal plane. A 3D view of the airway can be readily available with CBCT imaging. Using CBCT images filtered to show airway, it is possible to quantify the volume of the airway and sinuses. The most constricted location of the airway can be found and the axial view of this region can be quantified. Orthodontists who are keenly interested in studying the patient's airway will surely continue to enhance the analyses that are available using the 3D information (Figs 6.4A to C). Also CBCT is now used to treat sleep apnea patients as assessment of complete air space volume measurement and volumetric analysis is possible.

Temporomandibular Joint Analysis

If temporomandibular joint (TMJ) disorders occur during development, they may alter the facial growth pattern and may also affect the growth of the ipsilateral part of the mandible with compensations in the maxilla, tooth position, occlusion and cranial base. CBCT allows the clinicians to assess and quantify these changes associated with TMJ disorders (Figs 6.5A and B).[3]

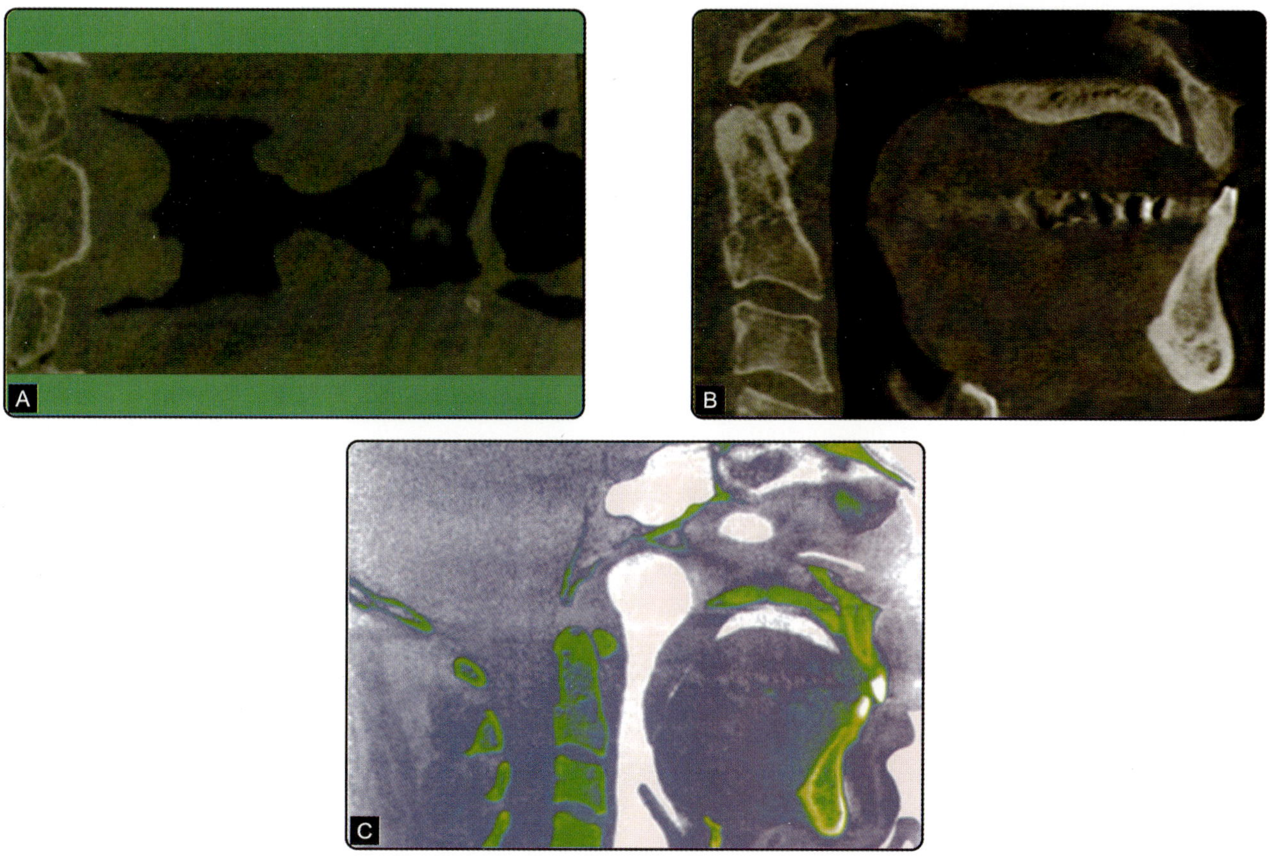

Figures 6.4A to C: Volumetric analysis of air space. **A.** Axial view; **B.** Sagittal view; **C.** Three-dimensional view.

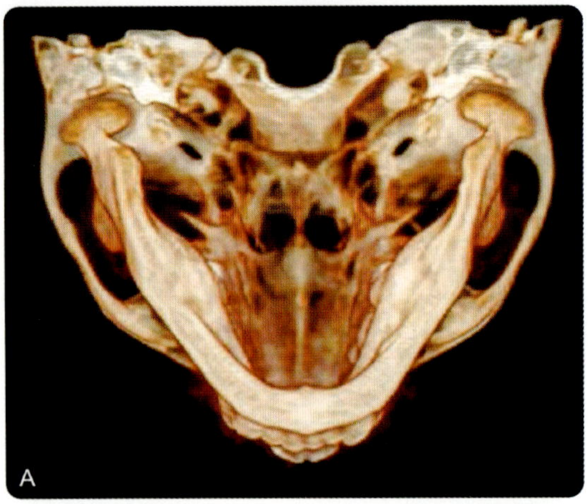

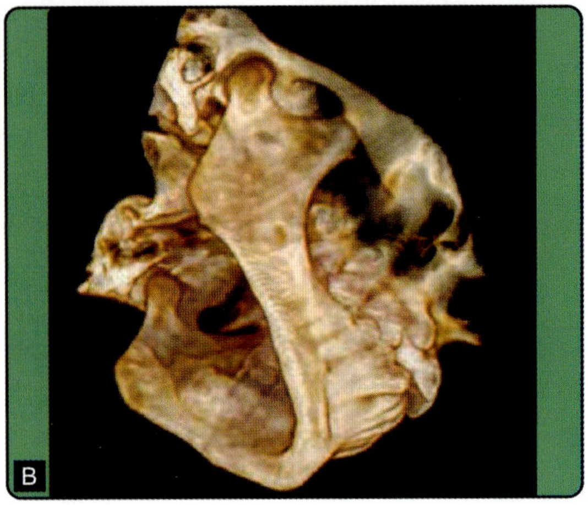

Figures 6.5A and B: Volume rendered image of temporomandibular joint (TMJ) through cone beam computed tomography (CBCT). **A.** Axial view; **B.** Lateral view.

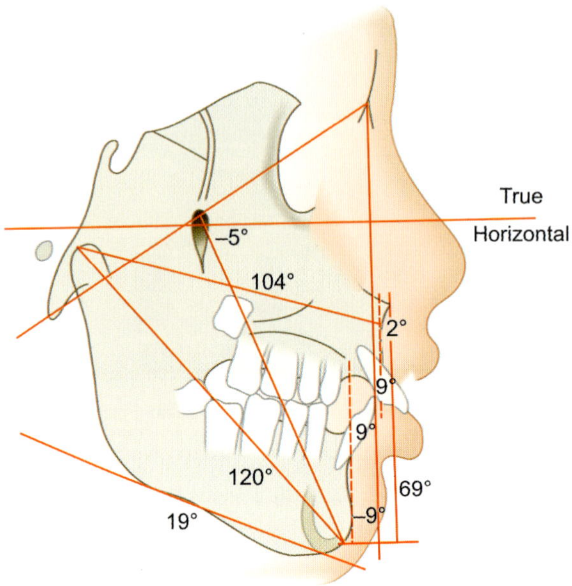

Figure 6.6: Metric method—use of selected linear and angular measures

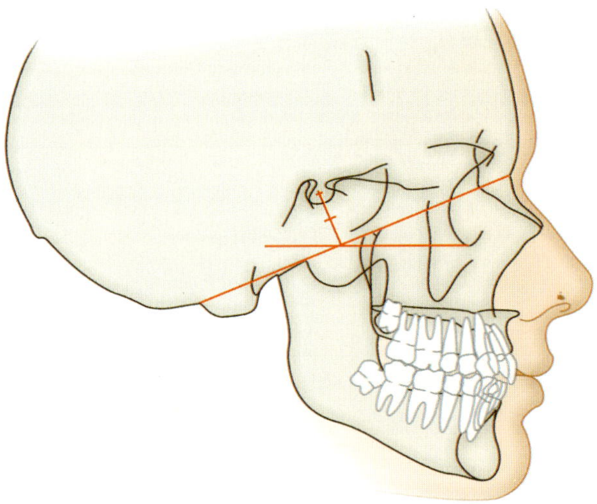

Figure 6.7: Graphic method—use of a composite template

Cephalometric Analysis

In orthodontics, the basic goal of cephalometric analysis is to assess the horizontal and vertical relationship of these functional components (Tables 6.1 and 6.2). There are two methods of cephalometric analysis:

1. Metric approach: Use of selected linear and angular measurements to establish appropriate comparisons. (Fig. 6.6).
2. Template analysis.

Identification of anatomic landmarks: Stable reference structures and maxillary, mandibular skeletal and dental. Graphically relating the dentofacial elements to these reference structures—'overlay' of individual's tracing on a reference template and visual inspection of degree of variation (Fig. 6.7).

The landmarks for cephalometric analysis must be located from whichever viewpoint as exact points and with a unique anatomical location and must be defined for each of the 3D spatial planes as coordinates.[14]

The various cephalometric analysis used in routine dental practice are:

- Down's
- Steiner's

- Tweed's
- McNamara's
- Burstone's.

Current 3D records are very useful, especially to accurately locate bilateral and transversal points that are better observed from the coronal plane. In this way it is possible to study and analyse, in greater depth and reliability, dentofacial asymmetries, problems on the transversal level of the maxillary bone structures, as well as the size of the structures that are involved in the skull.[16]

Table 6.1: Cephalometric analysis[15]

1. Skeletal	Norms	Preoperative	Postoperative
SN[*]	4–6		
Saddle angle	129 ± 5		
NS-Ar[†]			
S-Ar-Go[‡]			
A-Go-Me[§]			
Ar-Go-N[‖]			
N-Go-Me[¶]			
Y-axis	59.62 ± 3.09		
FMA[**]	23.83 ± 4.18		
SNA[††]	81.68 ± 2.37		
SNB[‡‡]	78.57 ± 2.81		
ANB[§§]	3.12 ± 1.81		
Facial angle	86.63 ± 3.02		
Pg to NB[‖‖] (mm)	2.13 ± 0.84		
AB plane	4.6 ± 3.67		
Angle of convexity	0.0 ± 5.09		
Wits appraisal			
Female	0.10 ± 1.77		
Male	1.17 ± 1.9		
2. Dental			
U Ins[¶¶] *(1)*			
1 to APg[***] (mm)	6.74 ± 1.32		
1 to NA[†††] (mm)	4.92 ± 2.05		
1 to NA (degree)	24.92 ± 5.82		
L Ins (1)			
1 to APg[‡‡‡] (mm)			
1 to NB[§§§] (mm)	6.00 ± 1.56		
1 to NM[‖‖‖] (degree)	27.88 ± 4.20		
IMPA[¶¶¶]	98.74 ± 4.39		
FMA[****]	23.83 ± 4.18		
FMIA[††††]	57		

Contd...

Contd...

	Norms	Preoperative	Postoperative
Interincisal Angle	123.86 ± 6.39	______	______
Cant of occlusal plane			
Skeletal to occlusal plane	66.90 ± 4.66	______	______
3. Soft tissue analysis			
E line U	______	______	______
E line L	______	______	______
S line U	______	______	______
S line L	______	______	______
Nosolabial angle	______	______	______

* SH/FH, sella-nasion/Frankfort horizontal plane; †NS-Ar, nasion articular; ‡S-Ar-Go, articular angle; §A-Go-Me, point-A-gonion-menton; ||Ar-Go-N, upper gonial angle; ¶N-Go-Me, nasion-gonion-menton; **FMA, Frankfort-mandibular angle; ††SNA, angle formed by sella nasion point A; ‡‡SNB, sella nasion point B; §§ANB, angle formed by point A nasion and point B; ||||Pg to NB, angle from pogonion and line extended from N to B; ¶¶U Ins, upper incisor; †††Ins, lower incisor; ‡‡‡APg, line extending from point A to nasion; §§§NB, line extending from point B to nasion; |||||| NM, line extending from nasion to menton; ¶¶¶IMPA, incisor mandibular plane; ****FMA, Frankfort mandibular angle; ††††FMIA, Frankfort-mandibular incisor angle.

Orthodontic Cephalometry[16]

Horizontal reference line: Constructed by drawing a line through nasion 7° up from sella-nasion line.

Table 6.2: Orthodontic cephalometry

Variables	Male norms	Female norms
Cranial base		
Ar-PTM* [horizontal plane (HP)] (mm)	37.1 ± 2.8	32.8 ± 1.9
PTM-N† (HP) (mm)	52.8 ± 4.1	50.9 ± 3.0
Horizontal (skeletal)	–	–
N-A-Pg‡ angle (degree)	03.9 ± 6.4	–2.6 ± 5.1
N-A§ (HP) (mm)	00.0 ± 3.7	–2.0 ± 3.7
N-B|| (HP) (mm)	–05.3 ± 6.7	–6.9 ± 4.3
N-Pg¶ (HP) (mm)	–04.3 ± 8.5	–6.5 ± 5.1
Vertical (skeletal, dental)	–	–
N-ANS** (HP) (mm)	54.7 ± 3.2	50.0 ± 2.4
ANS-Gn†† (HP) (mm)	68.6 ± 3.8	61.3 ± 3.3
PNS-N‡‡ (HP) (mm)	53.9 ± 1.7	50.6 ± 2.2
MP-HP§§ angle (degree)	23.0 ± 5.9	24.2 ± 5.0
Upper incisor-NF|||| (NF) (mm)	30.5 ± 2.1	27.5 ± 1.7
Lower incisor-MP¶¶ (MP) (mm)	45.0 ± 2.1	40.8 ± 1.8
Upper molar-NF (NF) (mm)	26.2 ± 2.0	23.0 ± 1.3
Lower molar-MP (MP) (mm)	35.8 ± 2.6	32.1 ± 1.9
Maxilla, mandible		
PNS-ANS (HP) (mm)	57.7 ± 2.5	52.6 ± 3.5
Ar-Go*** (linear) (mm)	52.0 ± 4.2	46.8 ± 2.5

Contd...

Contd...

Variables	Male norms	Female norms
Go-Pg[†††] (linear) (mm)	83.7 ± 4.6	74.3 ± 5.8
B-Pg[‡‡‡] (MP) (mm)	08.9 ± 1.7	7.2 ± 1.9
Ar-Go-Gn[§§§] angle (degree)	119.1 ± 6.5	122.0 ± 6.9
Dental		
OP[‖‖‖] upper-HP angle (degree)	06.2 ± 5.1	7.1 ± 2.5
OP lower-Hp angle (degree)	–	–
A-B[¶¶¶] (OP) (mm)	−01.1 ± 2.0	−0.4 ± 2.5
Upper incisor-NF angle (degree)	111.0 ± 4.7	112.5 ± 5.3
Lower incisor-MP angle (degree)	95.9 ± 5.2	95.9 ± 5.7

[*]Ar-PTM, linear distance between PTM point and nasion; [†]PTM-N, linear distance between PTM point and nasion; [‡]N-A-Pg, angle formed by nasion, point A and pagonion; [§]N-A, linear distance between nasion and point A drawn on horizontal plane; [‖]N-B, line joining nasion and point B; [¶]N-Pg, line extending from nasion and pogonian; [**]N-ANS, linear distance between nasion and anterior nasal spine; [††]ANS-Gn, linear distance between anterior and gnathion; [‡‡]PNS-N, linear distance between postnasal spine and nasion; [§§]MP-HP, mandibular plane-horizontal plane; [‖‖]NF, nasal floor; [¶¶]MP, mandibular plane; [***]Ar-Go, line extending from articular and gonion; [†††]Go-Pg, line extending from gonion to pogonion; [‡‡‡]B-Pg, line extending from point B to pogonion; [§§§]Ar-Go-Gn, gonial angle formed by articular gonion and gnathion.

The three spatial axes of importance in cephalometric analysis are (Figs 6.8 to 6.10):

1. Midsagittal plane (XZ): Anteroposterior vertical plane that divides the body in two halves (right and left portions), defined by the points Na, S, Ba, points of high reliability and of easy location.
2. Horizontal or transverse plane (XY): Horizontal plane perpendicular to the median sagittal plane that divides the body into upper and lower halves. We can obtain it and make it pass through each point that we choose, for example, through Na.
3. Coronal or frontal plane (YZ): Vertical plane perpendicular to the two previous ones that goes from one side of the body to another dividing it into two parts (anterior and posterior). It cuts through the midsagittal plane in the middle.

Orthognathic Surgery

Several applications of CBCT in orthognathic surgery treatment simulation, guidance and outcome assessment have been developed. CBCT 3D surface reconstructions of the jawbones are used for preoperative surgical planning and

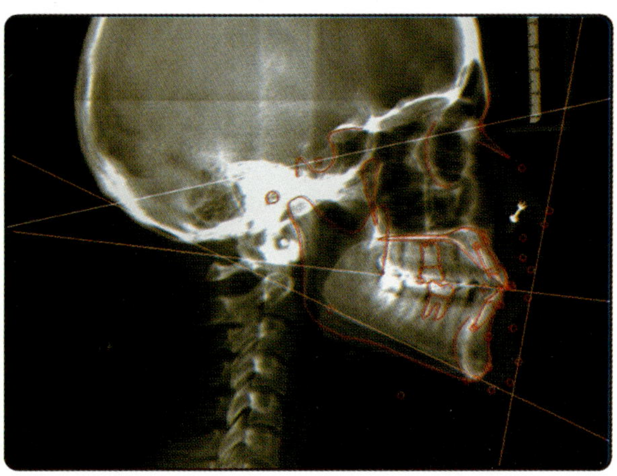

Figure 6.8: Steiner's analysis on cone beam computed tomography (CBCT) generated lateral cephalograph

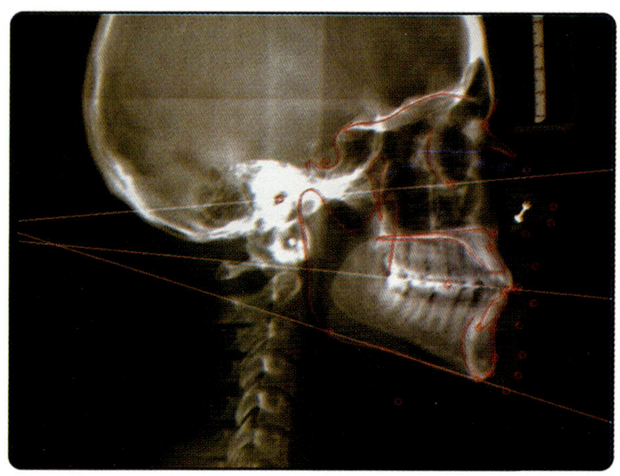

Figure 6.9: Tweed's analysis on cone beam computed tomography (CBCT) generated lateral cephalograph

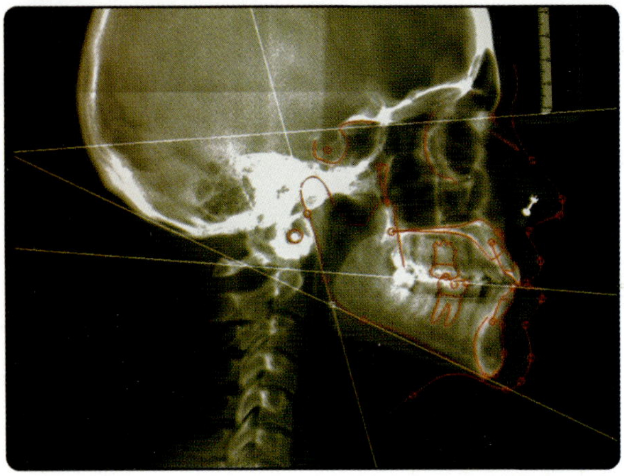

Figure 6.10: Burstone analysis on cone beam computed tomography (CBCT) generated lateral cephalograph

simulation in patients with traumas and skeletal malformations. Coupled with dedicated software tools, simulations of virtual repositioning of the jaws, osteotomies, distraction osteogenesis and other interventions can now be successfully implemented. Pre- and post-operative 3D CBCT skull models can also be registered (i.e. superimposed on each other) to assess the amount and position of alterations in the mandibular rami and condylar head following orthognathic surgery of the maxilla and the mandible.

Three-dimensional reconstructions of the jawbones from CBCT are of sufficient quality for clinical work. However, 3D models of the dentition still suffer from deformations due to streak artifacts caused by metal fillings, crowns and bridges, orthodontic brackets, and other metallic dental appliances. Therefore, virtual 3D models of the dentition are obtained by scanning the dental cast using a high-resolution surface laser scanner. Custom-made interocclusal wafers can also be scanned separately and then combined with CBCT 3D reconstructions of the jaws to create composite skull models. These 'double scanning' techniques have been successfully applied to patients with jaw asymmetry and in severe malocclusion cases.

Image-guided Surgery

Secondary correction of the craniofacial skeleton after traumatic injury is dependent on the restoration of the contour of adjacent fractured bony elements. In complex fractures, particularly mid- and pan-facial fractures, adjacent bone may be significantly fragmented, displaced, or even missing, leaving little guidance for the re-establishment of a 3D skeletal architecture. Bone grafting may also be indicated for severe injuries in which there is loss of bone or extensive comminution, while maxillofacial surgeons now have a choice of fixation schemes and rigid internal fixation devices such as locking plate screw and lag screw systems, their operative approach is usually dependent on preoperative 3D visualization of CT data and/or perioperative visual assessment of skeletal landmarks. Computer-aided surgery (CAS), also referred to as image-guided surgery (IGS), has been forwarded as the next process in assimilating CT data intraoperatively (Figs 6.11A to D). The aim of CAS is to visualize a surgical tool on a monitor in real time within the images of the patient to guide maxillofacial surgery for 'real-time' (i.e. intraoperative) localization of displaced facial skeletal segments during reduction and internal fixation. CAS is facilitated by image navigation systems that consist of a computer workstation, image processing software, a display monitor, a localization system and specialized, trackable instrumentation. The system tracks the actual movements of the surgical instruments, which are projected onto the preoperative image data set displayed on the system monitor. Several image-guidance tracking systems have been used in maxillofacial surgery [e.g. Innovated System Group (ISG) Viewing Wand, Mississauga, Ontario, Canada and Stryker-Leibinger STN-system, Freiburg, Germany].

The key to the system is the matching or 'registration' of preoperative CT or magnetic resonance (MR) image data (virtual) to the physical space occupied by the patient during surgery to provide localization of the surgical tools within the operative space. There are essentially two registration strategies, anatomical fiducial registration or extrinsic markers such as skin-affixed fiducials, bone-anchored markers and head frame-mounted reference points (autoregistration). The major potential advantage of CAS is that it may increase intraoperative patient safety by assisting the surgeon in navigating through complex anatomy that may be altered or obscured by trauma. The precise tracking of instruments allows the surgeon to avoid critical structures (e.g. the eyes) adjacent to the sinuses and to navigate precisely to the site of the fracture, thus increasing the probability of better surgical outcomes.[8]

Recommendations for Cone Beam Computed Tomography in Orthodontics[17]

The choice of modality used for imaging an orthodontic patient is based on clinical judgment as to whether the examination is likely to provide a clinical benefit for the patient as well as an assessment of the risk. Best practice in orthodontics requires a judicious approach to imaging

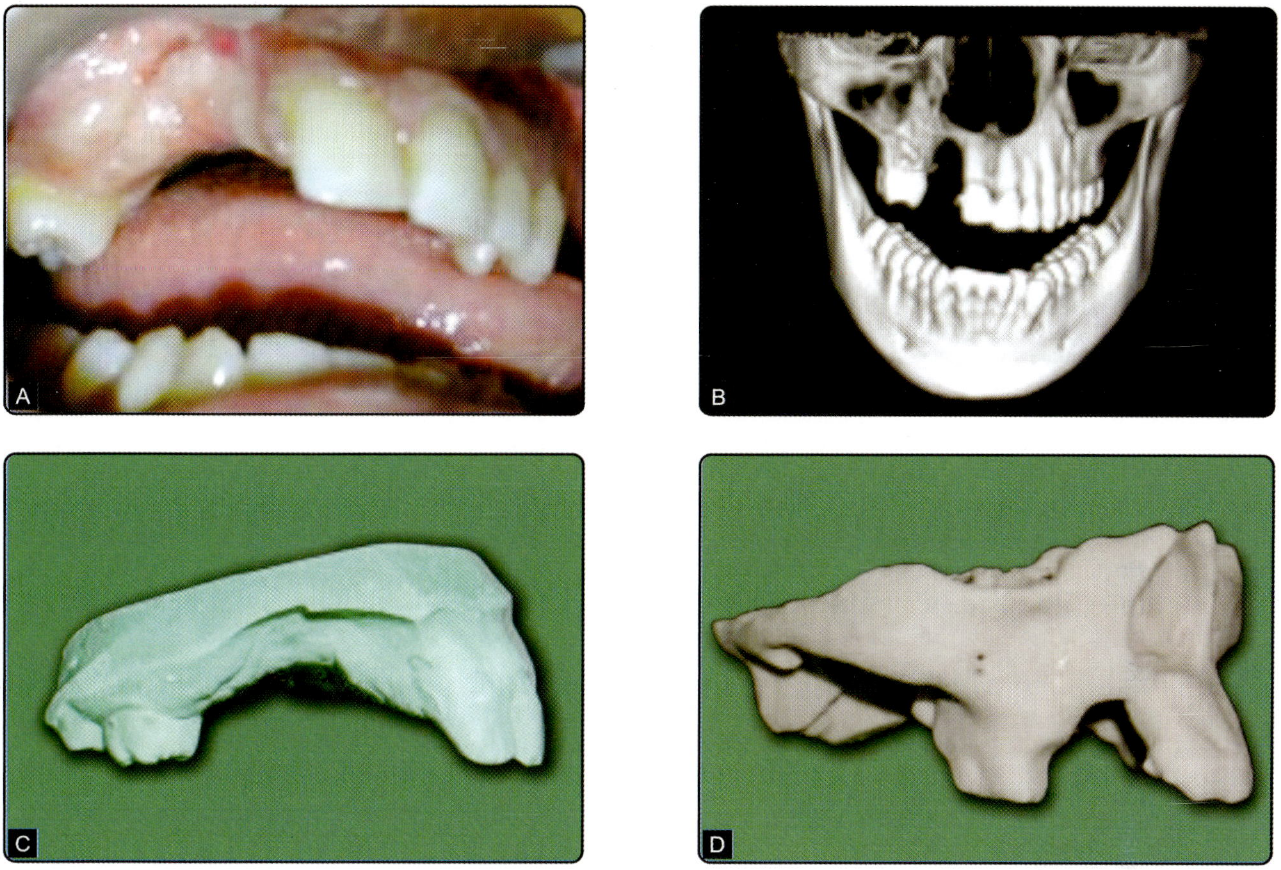

Figures 6.11A to D: Rapid prototyping models fabrication by cone beam computed tomography and stereolithography. **A.** Clinical picture; **B.** Computed tomography reconstruction; **C.** Patient cast model; **D.** Stereolithographic model.

Table 6.3: Consensus recommendations supporting the use of cone beam computed tomography (CTBD) imaging[17]

Recommendation	Consensus level	Definition
Likely appropriate	I	The use of CBCT imaging is indicated in most circumstances for this clinical condition; there is an adequate body of evidence to indicate a favorable benefit from the procedure relative to the radiation risk in the majority of situations
Possibly appropriate	II	The use of CBCT imaging may be indicated in certain circumstances for this clinical condition; there is a sufficient body of evidence to indicate a possible favorable benefit from the procedure relative to the radiation risk in many situations
Likely inappropriate	III	The use of CBCT imaging is not indicated in the majority of circumstances for this clinical condition; there is an insufficient body of evidence to indicate a benefit from the procedure relative to the radiation risk in most situations
Not supported	IV	The use of CBCT imaging has not demonstrated a consistent clinical benefit for this clinical condition and cannot be recommended at this time; there is either lack of weak or inconclusive body of evidence to indicate a benefit from the procedure relative to the radiation risk in this situation

based on the use of imaging selection criteria. These criteria are based on an appreciation of evidence-based benefits of the procedure and considerations for minimizing radiation risk. Imaging guidelines for the use of CBCT in contemporary orthodontic practice include (Tables 6.3 to 6.5):[17]

- Image appropriately according to clinical condition
- Assess the radiation dose risk
- Minimize patient radiation exposure
- Maintain professional competency in performing and interpreting CBCT Studies.

The American Association of Orthodontists (AAO) and American Academy of Oral and Maxillofacial Radiology (AAOMR) joint task force committee position statement provides both general recommendations and specific criteria for CBCT use based on specific clinical scenarios and most appropriate scan field of view.[17] The committee makes the following general recommendations for the use of CBCT in orthodontics.[17] The recommendations are as follows (refer Table 6.1):

1. Base the decision to order a CBCT scan on the patient's history, clinical examination and the presence of an appropriate clinical condition and assure the benefits to diagnosis and/or the treatment plan outweigh the potential risks of exposure to radiation, especially in the case of a child or young adult.
2. Use CBCT only when the clinical question for which imaging is required cannot be answered adequately by lower dose conventional dental radiography or alternate non-ionizing imaging modalities.
3. Do not use CBCT solely to facilitate the placement of orthodontic appliances such as aligners and computer bent wires or to produce virtual orthodontic models.
4. Design CBCT protocols to be task specific and to incorporate the imaging goal for the patient's specific presenting circumstances. The protocol includes considerations of exposure (mA and kVp), minimum, image-quality parameters (e.g. number of basis images, resolution), and restriction of the field of view (FOV) to visualize adequately the region of interest.
5. Do not perform a CBCT, if only 2D projected images derived from CBCT are to be used for diagnostic purposes.
6. Do not take a conventional image, if it is clear from the clinical examination that a CBCT study is indicated for proper diagnosis and/or treatment planning.

Table 6.4: Imaging selection criteria for the use of CBCT[*] in orthodontics[17]

Primary	Treatment difficulty	None	Dental structure anomalies	Anomalies in dental position	Compromised dentoalveolar boundaries	Asymmetry	Anterior posterior discrepancies	Vertical discrepancies	Transverse discrepancies	TMJ[†] signs and/or symptoms
Pretreatment	Mild	IV	FOVs[‡] (I)	FOVs (I)	FOVs, m (II)	FOVs, m (II)	FOVm,[§] l (II)	FOVm, l (II)	FOVm, l (II)	FOVs, m (III)
Moderate	FOVm, l (II)	–	FOVs (I)	FOVs (I)	FOVs, m (II)	FOVm, l (II)	FOVm, l (II)	FOVm, l (II)	FOVm, l (II)	FOVm, l (II)
Severe	FOVl[‖] (II)	–	FOVs[¶] (I)	FOVs[**] (I)	FOVs, m (II)[**]	FOVm, l (II)	FOVm, l (II)	FOVm, l (II)	FOVm, l (II)	FOVm, l (II)
During treatment	IV	–	FOVs[††] (III)	FOVs (II)	FOVs, m (II)	Presurgical FOVm, l (I)	Presurgical FOVm, l (II)	Presurgical FOVm, l (II)	Presurgical FOVm, l (II)	FOVm, l (II)
Post-treatment	IV[‡‡]	–	FOVs (III)	FOVs (III)	FOVs, m (III)	FOVm, l (II)	FOVm, l (II)	FOVm, (II)	FOVm, l (II)	FOVm, l (II)

[*]CBCT, cone beam computed tomography; [†]TMJ, temporomandibular joint; [‡]FOVs, small field of view; [§]FOVm, medium field of view; [‖]FOVl, large field of view; [¶]I, consensus recommendations; [**]II, likely appropriate; [††]III, likely inappropriate; [‡‡]IV, not supported.

Table 6.5: Definition of cone beam computed tomography (CBCT) field of view ranges for orthodontic Imaging[17]

Field of view	Abbreviation	Definition
Small	FOVs*	A region of radiation exposure limited to a few teeth or a quadrant within a dental arch, which include spherical volume diameters or cylinder heights ≤ 10 cm
Medium	FOVm†	A region of radiation exposure incorporating the dentition of at least one arch up to both dental arches, which include spherical volume diameters or cylinder heights > 10 cm and ≤ 15 cm
Large	FOVl‡	A region of radiation exposure incorporating anatomic landmarks necessary for quantitative cephalometric and/or airway assessment including the TMJ§ articulations with spherical volume diameters or cylinder heights > 15 cm

*FOVs, small field of view; FOVm†, medium field of view; FOVl‡, large field of views; §TMJ, temporomandibular joint.

Future of Cone Beam Computed Tomography in Orthodontics

As dentistry is moving into the digital realm, future uses for CBCT technology is constantly changing and new applications crop up almost daily.

Virtual Models

Plaster casts have been used in orthodontics for more than 100 years. They have been used to evaluate the patient's alignment, arch width and occlusion, tooth mass and soft tissue. Smaller voxel size and innovative software have led to the ability to reconstruct virtual orthodontic study models without the need to obtain alginate impressions. CBCT data can be used to produce 3D models without the need for alginate impressions.[18] These virtual models can be composed with or without roots evident. For many orthodontists, the presence of roots could be a major improvement over commonly used plaster casts, which only display the crowns. Also, these virtual models can be studied and measurements made on the computer. If 'hardcopy' models are needed, these can be fabricated from wax, starch, and plaster using rapid prototyping technology.[19]

Invisalign[3]

The Invisalign (Align Technology, Santa Clara, California) tooth movement system was introduced to orthodontics in 1999. A series of clear thermoplastic trays are used to gain the desired tooth movement. These removable, computer-generated trays are changed every 2 weeks until the desired alignment and occlusion are gained. Currently, the orthodontist supplies the Invisalign laboratory polyvinyl siloxane impressions and a bite registration. The laboratory uses a computer linked to a destructive scanner to assemble this information into 3D renderings of the patient's teeth. These virtual models are adjusted on a computer per the orthodontist's detailed prescription of tooth movement. Once approved, the computer images are converted to 'hardcopy' models using stereolithography and the clear trays are fabricated from these models.[20] It may be possible in the future to execute the entire fabrication process of the aligners using CBCT digital data. The CBCT images could be used to create the virtual models, thus negating the need to take and mail impressions, and a bite registration. This information could be transferred electronically to certain laboratories (e.g. Align Technologies) and the desired virtual tooth movement can be accomplished by way of e-mail communication between the orthodontist, and the laboratory. Even the retainers could be fabricated by the data in the laboratory computer database of the final tooth positions.

Insignia[3]

The Insignia process (Ormco Corporation, Orange, California) uses 3D imaging data and precision manufacturing to custom make orthodontic brackets and wires for an individual patient. Using an accurate impression taken by the orthodontist, the Insignia laboratory digitally constructs a virtual model of the teeth using specialized 3D scanners. Insignia software integrates these precision images with the orthodontist's prescription to calculate the optimum alignment and occlusion. The bracket for each tooth is then custom fabricated, taking into account the shape of the labial surface of the tooth and its root angulation and overall anatomy. An indirect bonding transfer mechanism is then fabricated, so that each bracket may be placed at a specific location on each individual tooth. Wires are fabricated by the laboratory to work closely with the custom brackets to supply the desired orthodontic tooth movement. It is anticipated that an accurate CBCT scan will replace the impression currently taken by the doctor. The treatment can be affected by patient motion and artifacts due to the CBCT scan. According to the manufacturer, the available software would require the CBCT data to have been acquired with a voxel size between 0.05 and 0.07 mm.

Suresmile[3]

Suresmile technology (OraMetrix, Inc. Richardson, Texas) uses the precision wire-bending capability of robots, combined with digital 3D scanning of teeth, computer simulation and special wire materials to facilitate orthodontic tooth movement in an accurate fashion. This system uses a handheld, 3D white-light scanning device to gain a virtual image of the patient's dentition. This procedure, done either through intraoral scanning or scanning of dental models, can be achieved with or without orthodontic brackets in place. These virtual images, along with the orthodontic prescription, are then used to position the dentition in its most aligned and interdigitated state. Wires are made by the Suresmile robot from a high technology and flexible material to reposition the teeth orthodontically to the desired occlusion and alignment. Additional scans are usually taken during treatment to refine the tooth movement. OraMetrix has been clinically beta testing the use of CBCT imaging to supply the virtual images of the teeth since the latter half of 2007. Voxel size of 0.2 mm or smaller is necessary to use this technology accurately. The accuracy of CBCT images in the Suresmile system again may be affected by patient motion and artifacts. Current software cannot adequately image all types of orthodontic brackets because of their composition. Plastic brackets seem to be the most difficult to visualize in CBCT scans. In the future, CBCT images could take the place of current orthodontic impressions and white-light scanning.

Orthodontic Temporary Anchorage Device Placement[3]

The temporary anchorage device (TAD) has gained popularity of late for use in orthodontic treatment. Many tooth movements that were mechanically difficult to accomplish in the past have become achievable with the use of these mini-implants. The knowledge of the root positioning can greatly enhance the opportunity for proper placement and success of TADs.[21] CBCT images allow more accurate and dependable views of the interradicular relationships than panoramic radiographs.[22] These images allow not only more successful placement but also better treatment planning of where these TADs should be placed, so that proper force vectors can be used during orthodontic treatment. CBCT data can be used to construct placement guides for positioning mini-implants between the roots of adjacent teeth in anatomically difficult sites.[23] The quality of the bone in the proposed placement sites can be evaluated before insertion of the mini-implants. Quantifying the thickness of the palatal bone can aid in determining the size and location of any TADs that may be treatment planned for the palate. CBCT images have been shown to be an accurate way to assess the volume of bone present at the proposed location.[24] The number of orthodontists using CBCT scans and TADs will increase significantly in the near future.

Software Advances[25]

For 3D cephalometry, the anatomical landmarks are identified on 3D surface-rendered volumes or models obtained from CBCT data. In the tracing step, cephalometric planes are defined using either three or four landmarks instead of the two landmarks traditionally used in 2D cephalometry. Beside the elimination of the superimposition of bilateral structures and unequal enlargement artifacts, this also allows for the evaluation of the right and the left sides of the skull independently. The quality and the visibility of the 3D cephalometric landmarks and parameters depend mainly on the scan field of view (FOV) selection, the 3D model segmentation threshold, and image artifacts.[26,27]

Three-dimensional Superimposition

One of the main advantages of the CBCT is that it allows superimposition of serial images to evaluate the growth and treatment changes. This is an efficient way for showing areas of bone displacement and remodeling, as well as demonstrating the changes in size, shape, and shift in positions of skeletal and soft tissues as a result of either orthodontic or surgical treatments.

The available software tools and options allow optimal alignment of the 3D CBCT datasets at different time points with high precision and accuracy after identification of specific anatomical landmarks, and structures. The computed registration is then applied to the segmented structures to measure changes due to orthodontic treatment or surgery. Surface distance calculations are then used for the purpose of accurate quantification of the changes or displacement due to either growth or treatment. Color mapping can show surface area distance differences between two 3D objects or 3D facial photographs.[28]

Three-dimensional Facial Photographs

One of the gold standard diagnostic tools in orthognathic surgery and preoperative orthodontic treatment is the 2D facial photographs that consequently reveal limitations in describing the 3D structures of a patient's face. CBCT and the newly introduced imaging techniques such as the 3D stereophotogrammetry (3D photographs) allows exploring the human face three dimensionally with multiple useful applications that ranges from using the facial scans to measure all the esthetic facial parameters to orthodontic diagnosis and evaluation of the craniofacial growth and development.[29]

Stereophotogrammetry is a method of obtaining an image by means of one or more stereo pairs of photographs being taken simultaneously. The 3D photography camera is used to capture the soft tissue surface of the face with correct geometry and texture information. The technique is based on the triangulation and fringe projection method. Image fusion (i.e. registration of a 3D photograph upon a CBCT) results in an accurate and photorealistic digital 3D data sct of a paticnt's facc.[30]

After registration or matching of the 3D photographs, the differences between the pre- and post-photographs can be visualized by a color scale or map. In this way, results of the treatment can be evaluated quantitatively and objectively. For clinical use, the registration process of pre- and post-treatment 3D photographs has to be very accurate.[31,32]

One of the recently introduced software features allow the facial photograph to be morphed onto a digital imaging and communications in medicine (DICOM) dataset where the 3D volume can generate a simulated 3D projection of the face in any frontal, lateral or user defined view of the face. By changing the translucency of the image, the correlation between the facial soft tissues to the skeleton can be determined. This has great implications in planning orthognathic surgery, orthodontic treatment, or other craniofacial therapies that could affect the facial appearance (Figs 6.12A to C and 6.13).[33,34]

The expanding use of CBCT technology is beneficial to both patients and practitioners, and is especially important to orthodontists because its ability to capture the entire anatomy needed for orthodontic treatment planning.[35] Craniofacial imaging is expected to become totally digital in the near future (refer Figs 6.11A to D). The continuous advancements in the imaging machines, techniques and software's have added valuable improvement in its diagnostic capabilities. When used correctly and responsibly, the data derived from CBCT imaging provides insight into treatment planning that is unachievable with other imaging methods and allows clinicians to provide more predictable patient care.

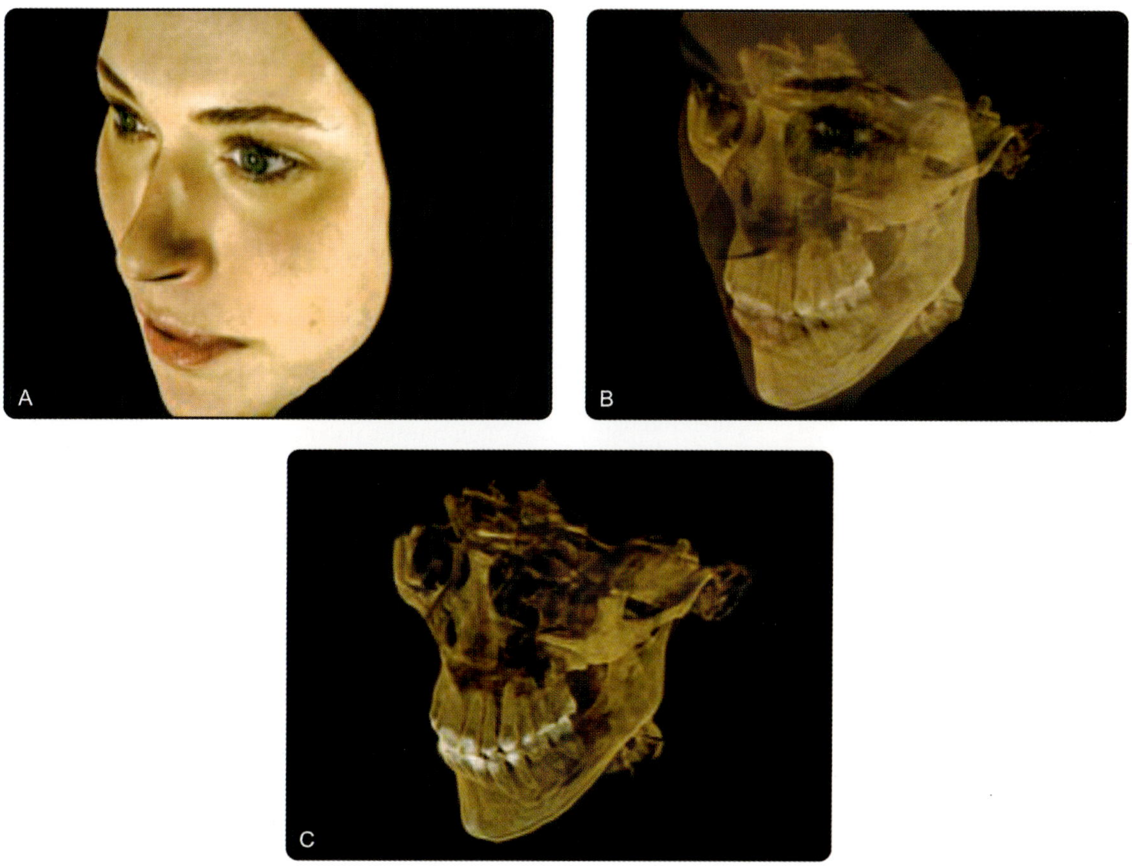

Figures 6.12A to C: Integrable face scanner (Galileos plus)

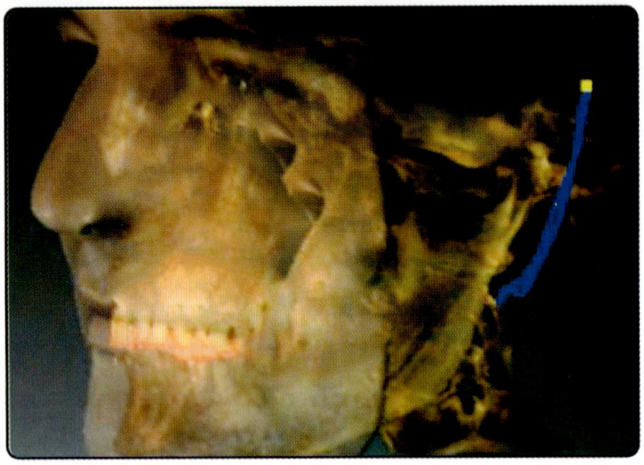

Figure 6.13: Integrated functional therapy (sicat function)

REFERENCES

1. Rakosi T. Cephalometry and radiographic analysis. In: Carruthers GB (Ed). An Atlas and Manual of Cephalometric Radiography, 1st edition. London: Wolfe Medical Publications Ltd; 1982. p. 7.
2. Steiner C. Cephalometrics for you and me. Am J Orthod. 1953;39:729-55.
3. Steven L Hechler. Cone-Beam CT: applications in orthodontics. Dent Clin N Am. 2008;52(4):809-23.
4. Elefteriadis J, Athanasiou A. Evaluation of impacted canines by means of computerized tomography. Int J Adult Orthodon Orthognath Surg. 1996;11(3):257-64.
5. Stewart J, Heo G, Glover K, et al. Factors that relate to treatment duration for patients with palatally impacted maxillary canines. Am J Orthod Dentofacial Orthop. 2001;119(3):216-25.
6. Walker L, Enciso R, Mah J. Three-dimensional localization of maxillary canines with cone-beam computed tomography. Am J Orthod Dentofacial Orthop. 2005;128(4):418-23.
7. Herring J. The effectiveness of orthodontists and oral radiologists in the diagnosis of impacted maxillary canines. Am J Orthod Dentofacial Orthop. 2007;132(6):861.
8. Ericson S, Kurol J. Early treatment of palatally erupting maxillary canines by extraction of the primary canine. Eur J Orthod. 1988;10(4):283-95.
9. Lund H, Gröndahl K, Gröndahl HG. Cone beam computed tomography evaluations of marginal alveolar bone before and after orthodontic treatment. Combined with premolar extraction. European Journal of Oral Sciences. 2012;120(3):2011.
10. Ludlow J, Laster W, See M, et al. Accuracy of measurements of mandibular anatomy in cone beam computed tomography images. Oral Surg Oral Med Oral Pathol Oral Radiol Endod. 2007;103(4):534-42.
11. Ceroni Compadretti G, Tasca I, Alessandri-Bonetti G, et al. Acoustic rhinometric measurements in children undergoing rapid maxillary expansion. Int J Pediatr Otorhinolaryngol. 2006;70(1):27-34.
12. Battagel J, L'Estrange PR. The cephalometric morphology of patients with obstructive sleep apnoea. Eur J Orthod. 1996;18(6):557-69.
13. Athanasiou AE, Papdopoulos M, Mazaheri M, et al. Cephalometric evaluation of pharynx, soft palate, adenoid tissue, tongue and hyoid bone following the use of a mandibular repositioning appliance in obstructive sleep apnea patients. Int J Adult Orthodon Orthognath Surg. 1994;9(4):273-83.
14. Zamora N, José-María Llamas, Rosa Cibrián, et al. A study on the reproducibility of cephalometric landmarks when undertaking a three-dimensional (3D) cephalometric analysis. Med Oral Patol Oral Cir Bucal. 2012;17(4):e678-88.
15. Chandrani. Roentgenographic Cephalometric Study of North Indian Children and Permanent Dentition. M.D.S. Thesis, PGI, Chandigarh. 1982.
16. Burstone CJ, James RB, Legan H. Cephalometrics for orthognathic surgery. J Oral Surg. 1978;36(4):269-77.
17. American Academy of Oral and Maxillofacial Radiology. Clinical recommendations regarding use of cone beam computed tomography in orthodontics. Position statement by the American Academy of Oral and Maxillofacial Radiology. Oral Surg Oral Med Oral Pathol Oral Radiol. 2013;116(2):238-57.
18. Mah J. The evolution of digital study models. J Clin Orthod. 2007;4(9):557-61.
19. Macchi A, Carrafiello G, Cacciafesta V, et al. Three-dimensional digital modeling and set up. Am J Orthod Dentofacial Orthop. 2006;129(5):605-10.
20. Wong B Invisalign A to Z. Am J Orthod Dentofacial Orthop. 2002;121(5):540-1.
21. Kuroda S, Yamada K, Deguchi T, et al. Root proximity is a major factor for screw failure in orthodontic anchorage. Am J Orthod Dentofacial Orthop. 2007;131(4 Suppl):S68-73.
22. Peck J, Sameshima G, Miller A, et al. Mesiodistal root angulation using panoramic and cone beam CT. Angle Orthod. 2007;77(2):206-13.
23. Kim S, Choi Y, Hwang E, et al. Surgical positioning of orthodontic mini-implants with guides fabricated on models replicated with cone-beam computed tomography. Am J Orthod Dentofacial Orthop. 2007;131(4 Suppl):S82-9.
24. King K, Lam E, Faulkner M, et al. Vertical bone volume in the paramedian palate of adolescents: a computed tomography study. Am J Orthod Dentofacial Orthop. 2007;132(6):783-8.
25. Ahmed Ghoneima, Eman Allam, Katherine Kula (2012). Three-dimensional imaging and software advances in orthodontics, orthodontics-basic aspects and clinical considerations. Farid Bourzgui (Ed). InTech. [online]. Available from: www.intechopen.com/books/orthodontics-basic-aspects-and-clinical-considerations/three-dimensional-3d-imaging-and-software-advances-in orthodontics.
26. Swennen G, Schutyser F. Three-dimensional cephalometry: spiral multi-slice vs cone-beam computed tomography. Am J Orthod Dentofac Orthop. 2006;130(3):410-16.

27. Halazonetis DJ. From 2-dimensional cephalograms to 3-dimensional computed tomography scans. Am J Orthod Dentofac Orthop. 2005;127(5):627-37.
28. Cevidanes L, Bailey L, Tucker GR, et al. Superimpositon of 3D cone-beam CT models of orthognathic surgery patients. Dentomaxillofac Radiol. 2005;34(6):369-75.
29. Lane C, Harrell W Jr. Completing the 3-dimensional picture. Am J Orthod Dentofac Orthop. 2008;133(4):612-20.
30. Maal T, Plooij J, Rangel F, et al. The accuracy of matching three-dimensional photographs with skin surfaces derived from cone-beam computed tomography. J Oral Maxillofac Surg. 2008;37:641-6.
31. Metzger MC, Hohlweg-Majert B, Schön R, et al. Verification of clinical precision after computer-aided reconstruction in craniomaxillofacial surgery. Oral Surg Oral Med Oral Pathol Oral Radiol Endod. 2007;104(4):e1:10.
32. Maal TJ, Loon B, Plooij J, et al. Registration of 3-dimensional facial photographs for clinical use. J Oral Maxillofac Surg. 2010;68(10):2391-401.
33. Harrell W. 3D diagnosis and treatment planning in orthodontics. Semin Orthod. 2009;15:35-41.
34. Schendel S, Lane C. 3D orthognathic surgery simulation using image fusion. Semin Orthod. 2009;15:48-56.
35. Ballrick JW, Palomo JM, Ruch E, et al. Image distortion and spatial resolution of a commercially available cone-beam computed tomography machine. Am J Orthod Dent facial Orthop. 2008;134(4):573-82.

7
Chapter
Role of Cone Beam Computed Tomography in Endodontics and Caries Diagnosis

Sushma P Jaju

INTRODUCTION

Radiography is essential to successful diagnosis of odontogenic and non-odontogenic pathoses, treatment of the pulp chamber and canals of the root of a compromised tooth via intracoronal access, biomechanical instrumentation, final canal obturation and assessment of healing. Imaging serves at all stages in endodontics.[1]

Preoperative stage imaging is required to assess the dental and alveolar hard tissue morphology and pathologic alterations to assist correct diagnosis. Intraoperative stage working length determination and 'master cone' selection radiography is essential. Postoperative stage final confirmation of outcome of treatment is evaluated on radiographs. Kells first reported the use of lead wire in root canal space on a 'radiogram' in 1899.[2-4]

Since then radiology has always played a pivotal role in the field of endodontics. Now century later with building on the pioneering efforts of those using conventional computed tomography (CT) and micro-computed tomography, the introduction of maxillofacial cone beam computed tomography (CBCT) in 1996 provided the first clinically practical technology demonstrating application of three-dimensional (3D) imaging for endodontic considerations.[1]

This new ability to image in the 3D dimension has created a paradigm shift for clinicians all around the world. CBCT imaging is slowly becoming the gold standard in an evidence-based approach to diagnosis, treatment planning and in delivering optimal care to the patients.

CONE BEAM COMPUTED TOMOGRAPHY IN ENDODONTICS

In endodontics, a machine with limited fields of view (FOV) should suffice. In general, the smaller the scan volume, the higher the spatial resolution of the image. As the earliest sign of periapical pathology is discontinuity in the lamina dura and widening of the periodontal ligament space, it is desirable that the optimal resolution of any CBCT imaging system used in endodontics does not exceed 200 µm—the average width of the periodontal ligament space.[5-8] The 3D Accuitomo (J Morita, Corporation, Kyoto, Japan) is the first of the small FOV systems, provided a resolution of 0.125 mm. Orthophos XG 3D (Sirona, Germany) is also providing a small FOV of 5 × 5 cm specifically for endodontic purpose (Fig. 7.1).

Assessment of Root Canal Morphology

The success of endodontic treatment depends on the identification of all root canals so that they can be accessed, cleaned, shaped and obturated.[9] The prevalence of a mesiobuccal (MB2) canal in maxillary first molars has been reported to vary from 69% to 93% depending on the study method employed. This variability occurs in the buccolingual plane where superimposition of anatomic structures impedes detection of small structural density changes.[10,11] Conventional radiographic techniques, at best, can only

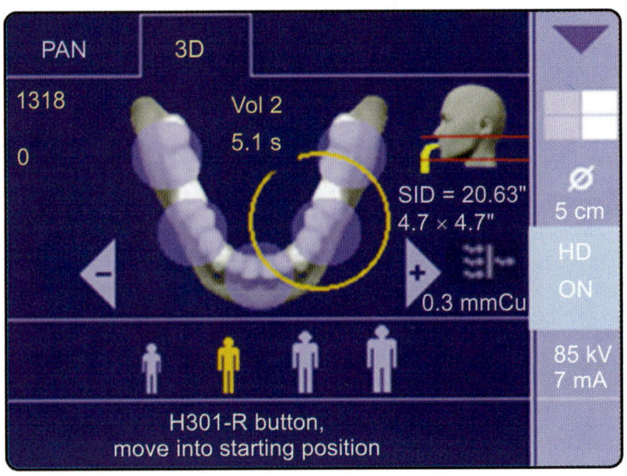

Figure 7.1: Fields of view of 5 × 5 cm volume for endodontic purpose

detect up to 55% of these configurations.[12] Ramamurthy et al and Matherne et al have described the limitations of two-dimensional (2D) imaging in detection of MB2 canal (Figs 7.2A and B).[13]

Study conducted by Neelkantan et al in Indian population revealed that the number of MB2 canal was more in maxillary first molar compared to second molar. Also type IV canal anatomy was more prevalent compared to Mongoloid population.[14]

Baratto Filho et al investigated the internal morphology of extracted maxillary first molars by comparing detection rates obtained using an operating microscope and CBCT to ex vivo sections.[15] They reported an ex vivo prevalence of a fourth canal in 67.14% of teeth and additional root canals in 92.85% of mesiobuccal roots. Clinical assessment provided slightly lower overall (53.26%), but higher (95.63%) MB2 detection rates whereas CBCT results showed the lowest overall (37.05%) detection rate. They indicated that CBCT provided a good method for the initial evaluation of maxillary first molar internal morphology, but that the use of operating microscopes was optimal. CBCT imaging has also been reported to characterize the high prevalence of the distolingual canal in Taiwanese individuals, highlight anomalies in the root canal system of mandibular premolars and assist in the determination of root curvature (Figs 7.3A to D and 7.4A to D).[16-18] With advent of newer software provided by CBCT companies like Orthophos XG 3D/Galileos (Sirona,Germany) working length determination of the root canal can be performed. But its validity and accuracy in clinical setup needs to be evaluated (Fig. 7.5).

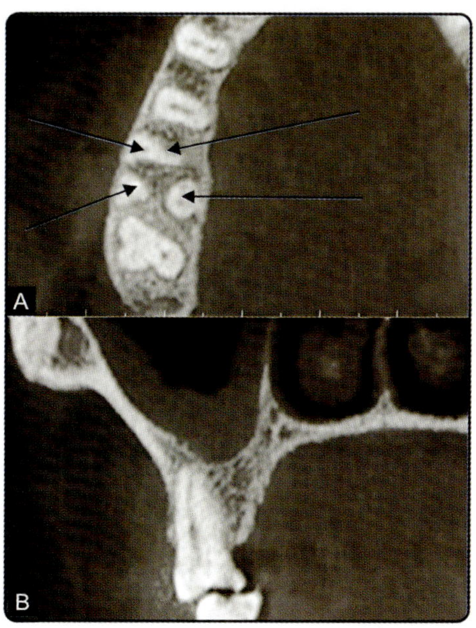

Figures 7.2A and B: Second mesiobuccal canal with right maxillary first molar. **A.** Axial view; **B.** Cross-sectional view

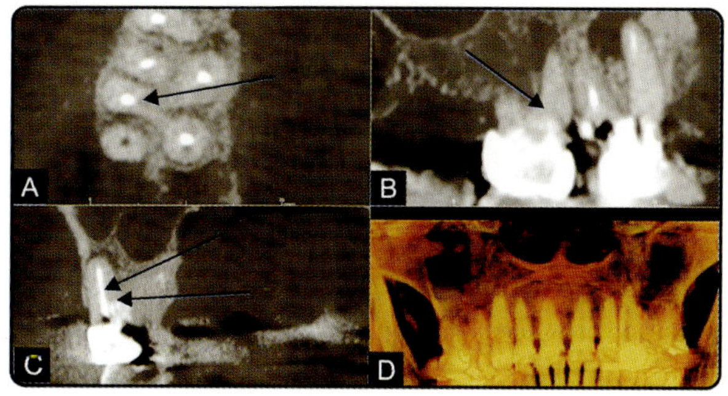

Figures 7.3A to D: Missed second mesiobuccal canal in maxillary right second molar leading to periapical infection

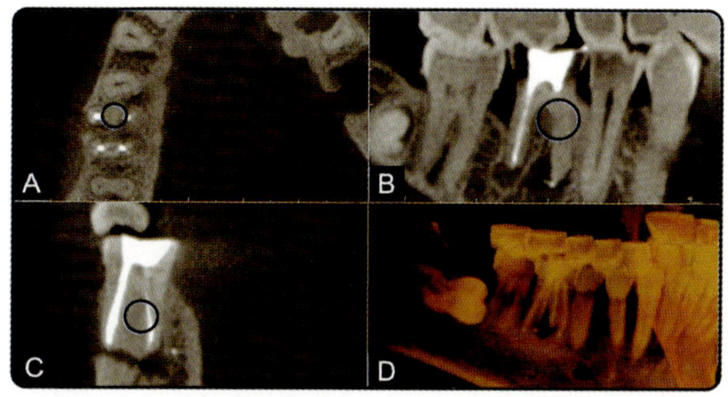

Figures 7.4A to D: Mesiobuccal and mesiolingual canal is filled, isthmus not cleaned properly leads to periapical infection

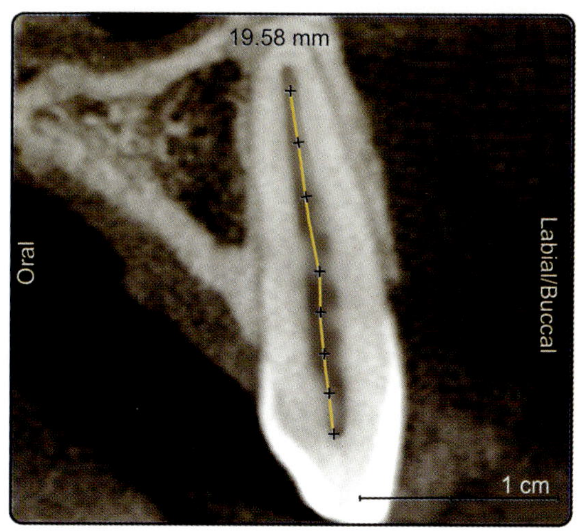

Figure 7.5: Root canal measuring tool (cross-sectional)

Dental Periapical Pathoses

The most common pathologic conditions that involve teeth are the inflammatory lesions of the pulp and periapical areas. CBCT technology now provides the clinician with the ability to observe an area in three different planes and thus acquire 3D information. Lesions confined to cancellous bone with little or no cortical plate erosion can be difficult to diagnose with intraoral film.[4] Lofthag-Hansen et al, Stavropoulos and Wenzel compared the accuracy limited FOV CBCT to intraoral radiographic paralleling technique.[1-19] They reported that CBCT provides greater diagnostic accuracy (61%) compared with digital (39%) and (44%) conventional radiographs. They indicated that, while detection rates for CBCT were higher, they did not advocate the replacement of intraoral radiography for detecting periapical lesions in routine clinical practice due to financial and dose considerations. Estrela and colleagues proposed a periapical index based on cone beam computed tomography periapical index (CBCTPAI) for identification of apical periodontitis (AP).[20]

The CBCTPAI is a 6-point (0–5) scoring system calculated from determining the largest lesional measurement in either the buccopalatal, mesiodistal or diagonal dimension and taking into account expansion, and destruction of cortical bone. The CBCTPAI is detailed in Table 7.1.

Table 7.1: Cone beam computed tomography periapical index score

Score	Quantitative bone alterations in mineral structures
0	Intact periapical bone structures
1	Diameter of periapical radiolucency > 0.5–1 mm
2	Diameter of periapical radiolucency > 1–2 mm
3	Diameter of periapical radiolucency > 2–4 mm
4	Diameter of periapical radiolucency > 4–8 mm
5	Diameter of periapical radiolucency > 8 mm
Score (n)	+E Expansion of periapical cortical bone
Score (n)	+D Destruction of periapical cortical bone

Using this periapical index, Low et al concluded that CBCT performed better in detection of periapical lesions compared with conventional imaging (Figs 7.6A and B).[21]

The CBCT technology and assignment of gray values might aid in the diagnosis of cyst versus granuloma.[4] The generally higher detection rates afforded by CBCT are similar to those reported for conventional CT.[22] This may be of clinical importance in patients, who complaints of pain or who have poorly localized symptoms associated with an untreated or previously root-treated tooth with no evidence of pathology identified by conventional imaging (Figs 7.7A to C).[23,24]

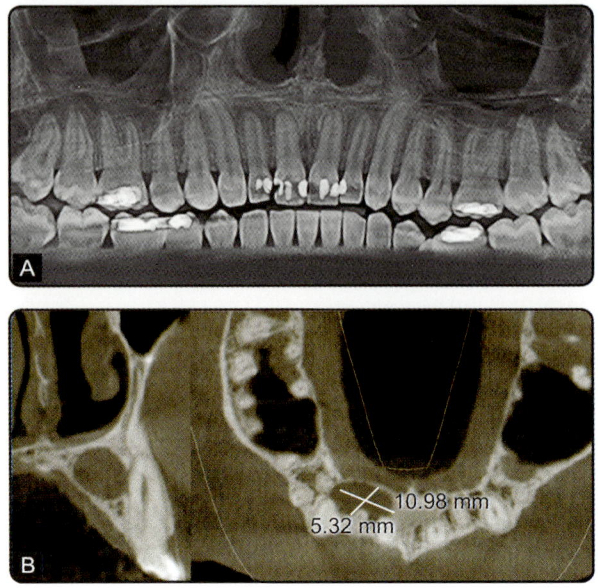

Figures 7.6A and B: Lateral variety of radicular cyst with right lateral incisor as seen on reconstructed orthopantogram (OPG). **A.** Reconstructed OPG; **B.** Cross-sectional and axial view.

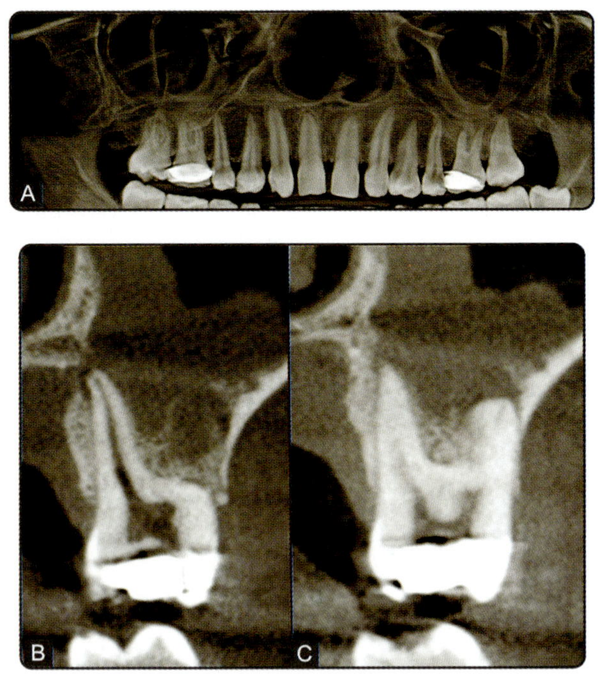

Figures 7.7A to C: Periapical lesion with maxillary right first molar extending into the maxillary sinus resulting in sinus inflammation. **A.** Reconstructed orthopantogram; **B** and **C.** Cross-sectional view.

Root Fractures

Usefulness and importance of CBCT in the diagnosis and management in specific aspects of dentoalveolar trauma, especially, root fractures, luxation and/or displacement and alveolar fracture has been studied extensively.[25-27] CBCT has found particular application for the diagnosis of root fractures (Figs 7.8A to C and 7.9A to D). Superiority of CBCT in detection of vertical and horizontal root fractures has been described in literature.[28,29] Elimination of superimposition of anatomic structures allows the clinician to analyze the fracture clearly. In addition, a 3D reconstruction can be fabricated of both the tooth and alveolar bone.[4] CBCT is the preferred modality of diagnosis of root fractures, which could be missed in conventional imaging techniques (Figs 7.10A to E).

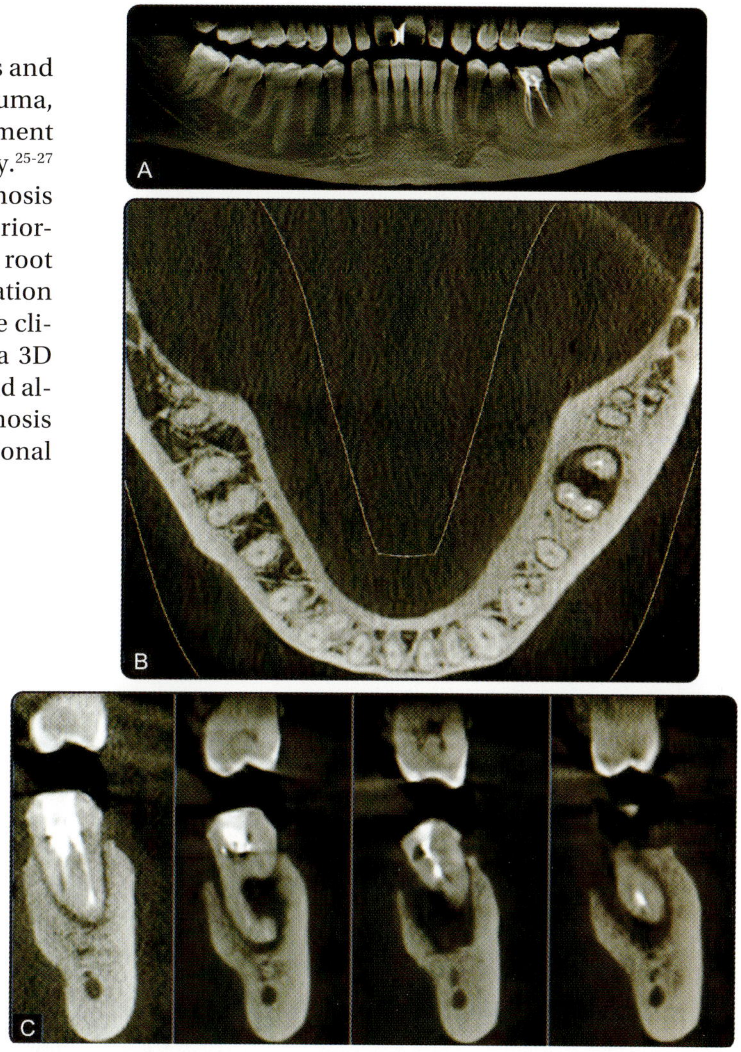

Figures 7.8A to C: Endodontic periodontal lesion with mandibular left first molar seen on cone beam computed tomography images. **A.** Reconstructed orthopantogram; **B.** Axial view; **C.** Cross-sectional view.

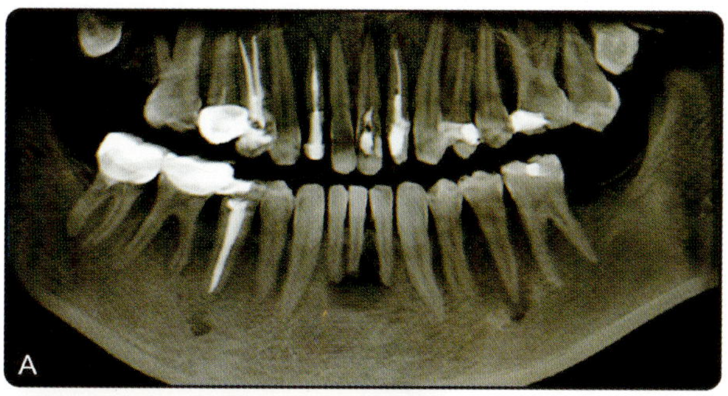

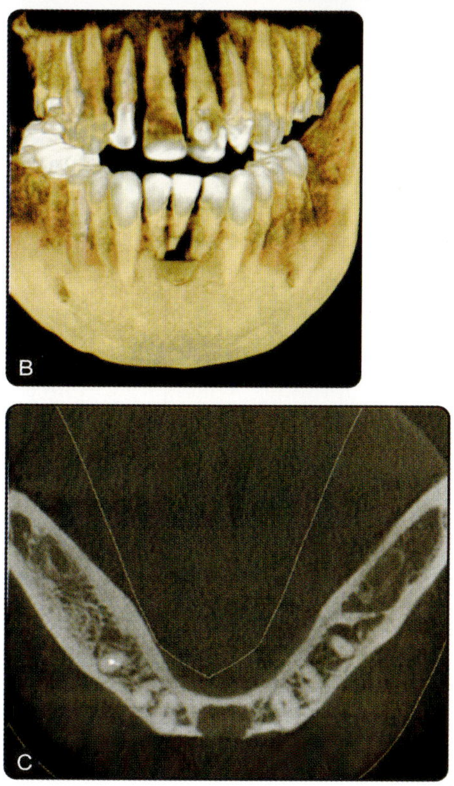

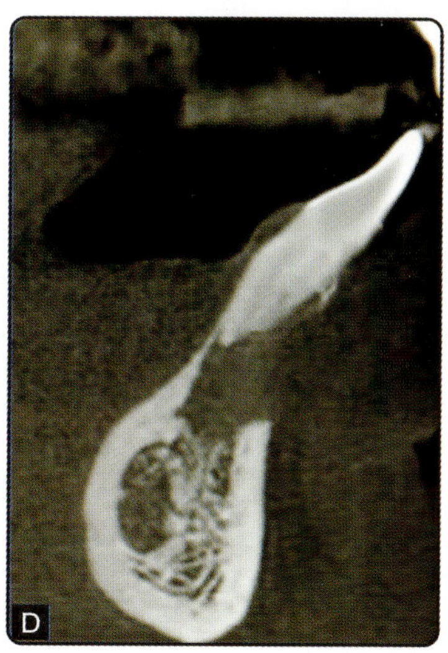

Figures 7.9A to D: Periapical infection causing thinning and loss of labial cortical plates in mandibular anterior region. **A.** Reconstructed orthopantogram; **B.** Three-dimensional reconstruction; **C.** Axial view; **D.** Cross-sectional view.

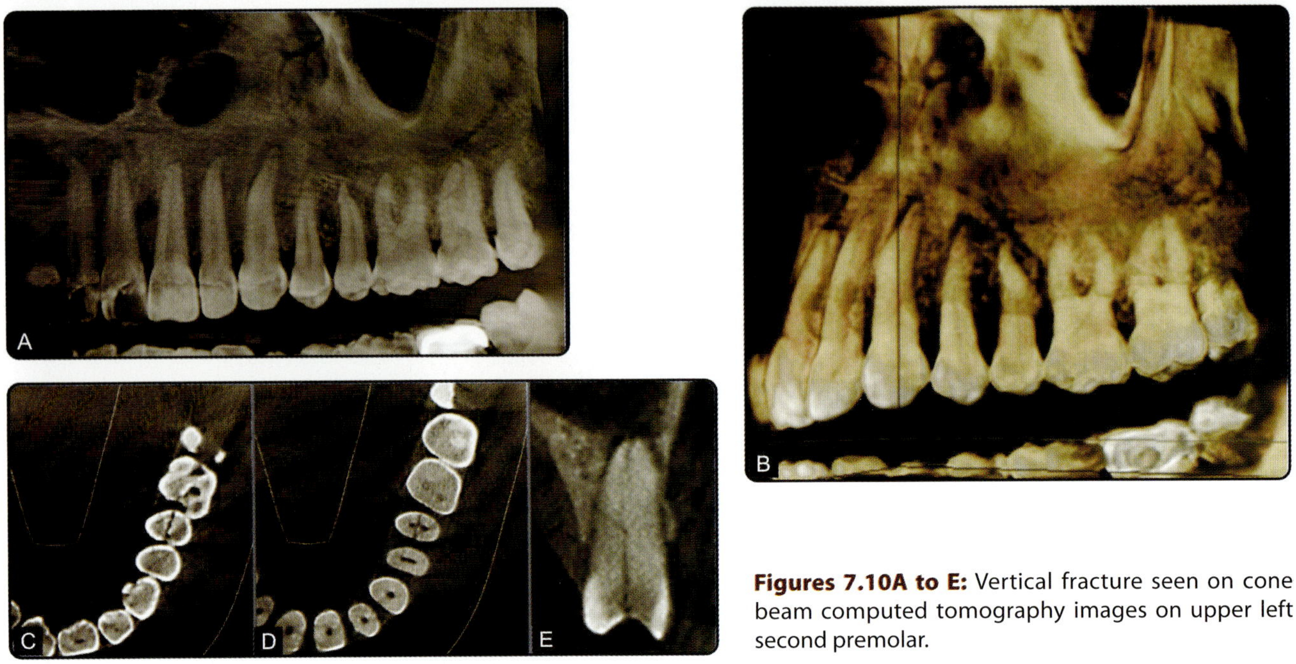

Figures 7.10A to E: Vertical fracture seen on cone beam computed tomography images on upper left second premolar.

Root Resorption

Root resorption is the loss of dental hard tissues as a result of clastic activities. It might occur as a physiologic or pathologic phenomenon.[30] Root resorption might be broadly classified into external or internal resorption by the location of the resorption in relation to the root surface. Compared with external root resorption, internal root resorption is a relatively rare occurrence, and its etiology and pathogenesis have not been completely elucidated.[31] The accuracy of CBCT in the detection of surface defects, while higher than conventional imaging modalities is not perfect and appears to increase with increasing voxel resolution of the volumetric dataset.[32] CBCT has also been shown to have particular application in the assessment of the postorthodontic apical root resorption and, in particular, of the roots of lateral maxillary incisors by impacted maxillary canines.[33-36]

On CBCT, external resorption presents with irregular radiolucency and intact root canal, internal resorption has clearly defined borders with no canal radiographically visible in the defect.[37]

The CBCT has been used successfully to confirm the presence of internal root resorption and differentiate it from external root resorption.[38] Conventional radiography is often unable to identify the true extent, location or the portal entry of a resorptive lesion. CBCT has been shown to help determine treatment complexity as well as aid the clinician in offering an accurate prognosis on the basis of the extent of the resorptive lesion. As a result of treatment and its outcomes are likely to become more predictable.[4]

Postoperative Assessment

Monitoring the healing of apical lesions is an important aspect of postoperative assessment in endodontics.[1] Similarly, adequacy of root canal obturation is an important determinant of endodontic success, it might be considered that CBCT is used in the initial and subsequent monitoring of the integrity of root canal fillings.

Sogur et al reported that images acquired from phosphor plates and conventional films were better compared to CBCT images as presence of streaking artifacts from the gutta percha and sealer compromising the quality of those images as regards root filling evaluations.[39] CBCT can be used to analyze voids in root fillings. Voids larger than 30 μm are detected easily on CBCT images. For small void detection, all digital intraoral techniques performed better than CBCT images.

The utility of CBCT in determining the precise nature of a perforation and the role of this on subsequent treatment has been illustrated by Young (Fig. 7.11).[40]

Preoperative assessment of periapical surgery site is of utmost importance to avoid postoperative complications. Proximity to mandibular canal, mental foramen and maxillary sinus during periapical surgery can be assessed accurately on CBCT images. Rigolone et al first described the value of CBCT in planning for endodontic surgery.[41]

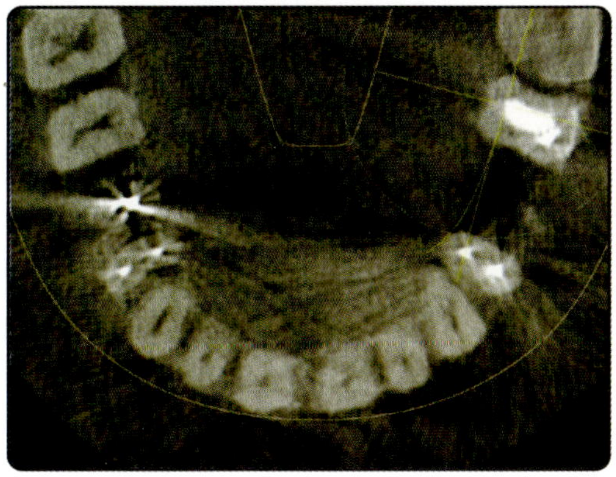

Figure 7.11: Root canal obturation artifact

The importance of CBCT for apical surgery of teeth adjacent to the maxillary sinus has subsequently been illustrated by Nakata et al who presented a case report localizing the presence of a periradicular lesion to a specific root and Tsurumachi and Honda who described the use of CBCT in localizing a fractured endodontic instrument protruding into the maxillary sinus prior to periapical surgery.[42,43]

Fractured Instruments

The CBCT provides information in all planes (coronal, sagittal, axial and cross-sectional) and hence this inherent advantage is utilized for locating fractured or separated root canal instruments within the root canal. Correct identification, precise location and length of separated instrument can be preoperatively determined, and later this information could be used for removal of the separated instrument.

Calcified Canals

When canals are identified, but are subjected to calcification, intraoperative CBCT has been shown to be a powerful tool for assessing the extent of calcification, thereby contributing to determining the proper sequence of the treatment. CBCT images permits the visualization of the depth of calcifications and guided the clinician to the correct location, angle and depth to access the patent portion of the canals. On the basis of accurate measurement of the length, width of canal walls and distance from important anatomic structures provided by the CBCT, the canals can be found, and properly treated. On the other hand, when complete calcifications were detected, the intraoperative CBCT provide the critical information that lead to the decision of preserving dental structures. Particularly, when apical pathosis is not present and the risks of attempting to expose a completely calcified canal are unjustifiable.

Recommendations of American Association of Endodontists for CBCT

In general, the use of CBCT in endodontics should be limited to the assessment and treatment of complex endodontic conditions such as:

1. Identification of potential accessory canals in teeth with suspected complex morphology based on conventional imaging.
2. Identification of root canal system anomalies and determination of root curvature.
3. Diagnosis of dental periapical pathosis in patients who present with contradictory or non-specific clinical signs and symptoms, who have poorly localized symptoms associated with an untreated or previously endodontically treated tooth with no evidence of pathosis identified by conventional imaging and in cases where anatomic superimposition of roots or areas of the maxillofacial skeleton is required to perform task-specific procedures.
4. Diagnosis of non-endodontic origin pathosis in order to determine the extent of the lesion and its effect on surrounding structures.
5. Intra- or post-operative assessment of endodontic treatment complications, such as overextended root canal obturation material, separated endodontic instruments, calcified canal identification and localization of perforations.
6. Diagnosis and management of dentoalveolar trauma, especially root fractures, luxation and/or displacement of teeth and alveolar fractures.
7. Localization and differentiation of external and internal root resorption or invasive cervical resorption from other conditions and the determination of appropriate treatment, and prognosis.

Although, CBCT technology has been in the market place for several years, it is still very expensive. This limits most of the clinicians to send their patients for CBCT scans and read by a dental radiologist. This follows the medical model of imaging. Most endodontic applications only require a small FOV (4 × 4 mm). Limiting the FOV not only reduces dosage, scan time and scatter artifacts but it also focuses the volume on structures familiar to dentists. The routine use of CBCT technology in endodontics is fast approaching, but astute clinician should recommend use of CBCT on proper clinical diagnosis and prudent judgment.

CONE BEAM COMPUTED TOMOGRAPHY IN CARIES DIAGNOSIS

Bitewing radiographs and intraoral periapical radiographs are the conventional imaging modalities for early and late caries diagnosis. Panoramic radiographs have a dubious clinical application for caries diagnosis. CBCT imaging appears to be the best prospect for improving the detection and depth assessment of caries in proximal and occlusal lesions. Recent work with benchtop-based local or limited CBCT lung pixels valves (LCT) systems has demonstrated the potential for caries detection and depth characterization by high-resolution systems.[25] All five studies used a benchtop CBCT system with a high resolution (40 mm pixel) charge-coupled device (CCD) detector and rotating turntable with a fixed anode intraoral radiograph source. They also used histologically generated ground truth and small sample sizes of 24–30 teeth. LCT images were presented in parasagittal (similar to the bitewing view) and axial planes were compared with bitewing radiographs. General linear model and receiver operating characteristic curves with analysis of variance methods were the statistical methods used. Kalathingal and colleagues found no difference in the detection of carious lesions, but did find that LCT was superior for caries depth assessment, although sensitivity increased and specificity showed no difference. The work performed by van Daatselaar and coworkers demonstrated the superiority of LCT images for caries detection, and noted that the number of source images could be as low as 14, a significant finding because a CCD detector was used for the study.[25]

Turning to clinical CBCT systems, Akdeniz and coworkers, Tsuchida and colleagues used a limited-volume CBCT (LCBCT).[44] Accuitomo device and compared in vitro CBCT results with either conventional film radiography or storage phosphor (SP) images. Akdeniz and colleagues, using 41 teeth, histologically verified ground truth and all image planes for viewing found that LCBCT was superior for caries depth assessment when compared with SP and film. These results corroborated the work of Kalathingal and colleagues.[44]

A most recent and thorough study using full-volume CBCT and LCBCT by Haiter-Neto, and colleagues compared the NewTom 3G system (AFP Imaging, Elmsford, New York) using three FOV (12, 9 and 6 inch), the Accuitomo LCBCT system (J Morita Manufacturing Corporation, Kyoto, Japan), Insight film (Eastman Kodak Company, Rochester, New York) and Digora SP (Soredex, Tuusula, Finland) images for the detection of approximal, and carious lesions. The results showed that the NewTom 12 inch and 9 inch images had significantly lower sensitivities than the Accuitomo systems, whereas the NewTom 9 inch and 6 inch images had significantly lower specificities than the insight film and Digora images. The Accuitomo images were determined to be no different from film or the Digora-based images. For occlusal surfaces, the Accuitomo presented a higher sensitivity than the other systems. Specificity and overall true score did not differ among the modalities for occlusal lesions.[25] The investigators concluded that the NewTom 3G system had a lower diagnostic accuracy for caries detection than the intraoral or LCBCT systems. The LCBCT systems were determined to be equal to the intraoral systems, but did score higher in detecting dentinal lesions. These results are not surprising, given the lower spatial resolution of the NewTom system and the higher signal to noise ratio of the LCBCT system.[25] Typically, the sensitivities were higher for the CBCT modalities, but specificities were less, suggesting that one of the limitations of caries detection with CBCT imaging maybe an increase in the number of false positives. Further studies are needed to evaluate CBCT for the detection of occlusal or pit and fissure caries, a task for which 2D imaging has been weak. In addition, the reader is reminded that in the in vitro studies mentioned earlier, intraoral 2D images were usually obtained under ideal geometry conditions with no closed contacts, cone cuts or projective distortions. The equivalence of CBCT scores to those of 2D imaging may, in the minds of some, demonstrate the superiority of the former system. At this time, the application of CBCT imaging to caries diagnosis is promising, with more research needed, especially in vivo investigations. In addition, with current technology, it is assumed that teeth with metal or even radiopaque restorations should not be considered for CBCT caries imaging.

CONCLUSION

Cone beam computed tomography is gradually expanding its role in the field of endodontics. It is working as an adjunct imaging modality in complicated cases, which are missed on conventional imaging.

REFERENCES

1. Scarfe WC, Levin MD, Gane D, et al. Use of cone beam computed tomography in endodontics. Int J Dent. 2009;634:56.
2. Langland OE, Langlais RP. Early pioneers of oral and maxillofacial radiology. Oral Surg Oral Med Oral Pathol Oral Radiol Endod. 1995;80(5):496-511.
3. Jacobsohn PH, Fedran RJ. Making darkness visible: the discovery of X-ray and its introduction to dentistry. J Am Dent Assoc. 1995;126(10):1359-67.

4. Cotton TP, Geisler TM, Holden DT, et al. Endodontic applications of cone-beam volumetric tomography. J Endod. 2007;33(9):1121-32.
5. Grondahl HG, Huumonen S. Radiographic manifestations of periapical inflammatory lesions. How new radiological techniques may improve endodontic diagnosis and treatment planning? Endodontic Topics. 2004;8:55-67.
6. Goldman M, Pearson AH, Darzenta N. Endodontic success—who's reading the radiograph? Oral Surg Oral Med Oral Pathol. 1972;33(3):432-7.
7. Leung SF. Cone Beam Computed Tomography in Endodontics. The HongKong Medical Diary. 2013;15(3):16-9.
8. Nesari R, Rossman LE, Kratchman SI. Cone-beam computed tomography in endodontics: are we there yet? Compend Contin Educ Dent. 2009;30(6):312-8.
9. Vertucci FJ. Root canal anatomy of the human permanent teeth. Oral Surg Oral Med Oral Patho. 1984;58(5):589-99.
10. Pineda F. Roentgenographic investigation of the mesiobuccal root of the maxillary first molar. Oral Surg Oral Med Oral Pathol. 1973;36(2):253-60.
11. Nance R, Tyndall D, Levin LG, et al. Identification of root canals in molars by tuned-aperture computed tomography. Int Endod J. 2000;33(4):392-6.
12. Ramamurthy R, Scheetz JP, Clark SJ, et al. Effects of imaging system and exposure on accurate detection of the second mesio-buccal canal in maxillary molar teeth. Oral Surg Oral Med Oral Patho Oral Radio Endod. 2006;102(6):796-802.
13. Matherne RP, Angelopoulos C, Kulild JC, et al. Use of cone-beam computed tomography to identify root canal systems in vitro. J Endod. 2008;34(1):87-9.
14. Neelakantan P, Subbarao C, Ahuja R, et al. Cone-beam computed tomography study of root and canal morphology of maxillary first and second molars in an Indian population. J Endod. 2010;36(10):1622-7.
15. Baratto F, Zaitter S, Haragushiku GA, et al. Analysis of the internal anatomy of maxillary first molars by using different methods. J Endod. 2009;35(3):337-42.
16. Tu MG, Huang HL, Hsue SS, et al. Detection of permanent three-rooted mandibular first molars by cone-beam computed tomography imaging in Taiwanese individuals. J Endod. 2009;35(4):503-7.
17. Cleghorn BM, Christie WH, Dong CC. Anomalous mandibular premolars: a mandibular first premolar with three roots and a mandibular second premolar with a C-shaped canal system. Int Endod J. 2008;41(11):1005-14.
18. Estrela C, Bueno MR, Sousa-Neto MD, et al. Method for determination of root curvature radius using cone-beam computed tomography images. Brazilian Dent J. 2008;19(2):114-8.
19. Lofthag-Hansen S, Huumonen S, Grondahl K, et al. Limited cone beam CT and intraoral radiography for the diagnosis of periapical pathology. Oral Surg Oral Medl Oral Pathol Oral Radio Endod. 2007;103(1):114-9.
20. Estrela C, Bueno MR, Azevedo BC, et al. A new periapical index based on cone beam computed tomography. J Endod. 2008;34(11):1325-31.
21. Low KM, Dula K, Burgin W, et al. Comparison of periapical radiography and limited cone-beam tomography in posterior maxillary teeth referred for apical surgery. J Endod. 2008;34(5):557-62.
22. Jorge EG, Tanomaru-Filho M, Gonalves M, et al. Detection of periapical lesion development by conventional radiography or computed tomography. Oral Surg Oral Med Oral Pathol Oral Radiol Endod. 2008;106(1):e56-61.
23. Grondahl HG, Huumonen S. Radiographic manifestations of periapical inflammatory lesions. How new radiological techniques may improve endodontic diagnosis and treatment planning. Endodontic Topics. 2004;8:55-67.
24. Patel S, Dawood A, Ford TP, et al. The potential applications of cone beam computed tomography in the management of endodontic problems. Int: Endod J. 2007;40(10) 818-30.
25. Tyndall DA, Rathore S. Cone-beam CT diagnostic applications: caries, periodontal bone assessment and endodontic applications. DCNA. 2008;52(4):825-41.
26. Cohenca N, Simon JH, Roges R, et al. Clinical indications for digital imaging in dentoalveolar trauma. Part 1: traumatic injuries. Dental Traumatology. 2007;23(2):95-104.
27. Ilguy D, Ilguy M, Fisekcioglu E, et al. Detection of jaw and root fractures using cone beam computed tomography: a case report. Dentomaxillofacial Radiology. 2009;38(3):169-73.
28. Hassan B, Metska ME, Ozok AR, et al. Detection of vertical root fractures in endodontically treated teeth by a cone beam computed tomography scan. J Endod. 2009;35(5):719-22.
29. Kamburoglu K, Ilker Cebeci AR, Grondahl HG. Effectiveness of limited cone-beam computed tomography in the detection of horizontal root fracture. Dental Traumatology. 2009;25(3):256-61.
30. Patel S, Ford TP. Is the resorption external or internal? Dent Update. 2007;34(4):218-29.
31. Patel S, Ricucci D, Durak C, et al. Internal root resorption: a review. J Endod. 2010;36(7):1107-21.
32. Hahn W, Fricke-Zech S, Fricke J, et al. Detection and size differentiation of simulated tooth root defects using flat-panel volume computerized tomography. Oral Surg Oral Med Oral Pathol Oral Radiol Endod. 2009;107(2):272-8.
33. Dudic A, Giannopoulou C, Leuzinger M, et al. Detection of apical root resorption after orthodontic treatment by using panoramic radiography and cone-beam computed tomography of super-high resolution. American Journal of Orthodontics and Dentofacial Orthopedics. 2009;135(4):434-7.
34. Walker L, Enciso R, Mah J. Three-dimensional localization of maxillary canines with cone-beam computed tomography. American Journal of Orthodontics and Dentofacial Orthopedics. 2005;128(4):418-23.
35. Liu DG, Zhang WL, Zhang ZY, et al. Localization of impacted maxillary canines and observation of adjacent incisor resorption with cone-beam computed tomography. Oral Surg Oral Med Oral Pathol Oral Radiol Endod. 2008; 105(1):91-8.

36. Hechler SL. Cone-beam CT: applications in orthodontics. DCNA. 2008;52(4):809-23.
37. Gulabivala K, Searson LJ. Clinical diagnosis of internal resorption: an exception to the rule. Int: Endod J. 1995;28(5):255-60.
38. Cohenca N, Simon JH, Mathur A, et al. Clinical indications for digital imaging in dento-alveolar trauma. part 2: root resorption. Dental Traumatology. 2007;23(2):105-13.
39. Sogur E, Baksi BG, Grondahl HG. Imaging of root canal fillings: a comparison of subjective image quality between limited cone-beam CT, storage phosphor and film radiography. Int: Endod J. 2007;40(3):179-85.
40. Young GR. Contemporary management of lateral root perforation diagnosed with the aid of dental computed tomography. Aust Endod J. 2007;33(3):112-8.
41. Rigolone M, Pasqualini MD, Bianchi L, et al. Vestibular surgical access to the palatine root of the superior first molar: 'low-dose cone-beam' CT analysis of the pathway and its anatomic variations. J Endod. 2003;29(11):773-5.
42. Nakata K, Naitoh M, Izumi M, et al. Effectiveness of dental computed tomography in diagnostic imaging of periradicular lesion of each root of a multirooted tooth: a case report. J Endod. 2006;32(6)583-7.
43. Tsurumachi T, Honda K. A new cone beam computerized tomography system for use in endodontic surgery. Int: Endod J. 2007;40(3):224-32.
44. Kalathingal SM, Mol A, Tyndall DA, et al. In vitro assessment of cone beam local computed tomography for proximal caries detection. Oral Surg Oral Med Oral Pathol Oral Radiol Endod. 2007;104(5):699-704.

8 Chapter

Role of Cone Beam Computed Tomography in Oral and Maxillofacial Pathologies

Prashant P Jaju

INTRODUCTION

Imaging plays an important role in oral and maxillofacial surgery diagnosis and treatment planning. A thorough history and clinical examination are vital in establishing diagnosis supported by radiographical examination. Two-dimensional (2D) projection radiography is traditionally being used for diagnosing congenital and developmental deformities in the maxillofacial region. Still, over the last few decades, the introduction of three-dimensional (3D) imaging characterized by computed tomography (CT) and magnetic resonance imaging (MRI) technologies has had a tremendous impact on the practice and teaching of maxillofacial surgery.[1]

Cone beam CT has fully demonstrated its role in the field of oral maxillofacial surgery, maxillofacial trauma, impaction, bony pathologies, cleft palate and temporomandibular disorders.

CBCT IN ORAL MAXILLOFACIAL SURGERY

Tooth Impaction

Surgical removal of impacted teeth demands precise knowledge of the tooth location in the jaw and its relation to other teeth and surrounding anatomical structures. For instance, in the mandible, the relationship of the roots of impacted third molars to the mandibular dental canal must be accurately assessed since the canal is frequently very closely associated with an impacted molar and postoperative complications due to nerve impingement are reported. It is necessary to assess whether a physical contact between the root and the border of the canal is present or not.[1]

Panoramic and/or intraoral radiographs are sufficient for preoperative imaging in most cases where there is no overlap between the inferior alveolar canal (IAC) and the lower third molar.[2] Kamrun et al revealed that the visibility of the superior border on panoramic images was very poor except for the most posterior area. The poor visualization of the canal on panoramic images was considered to be remarkably improved by the use of CBCT images.[3] Where impacted third molar is overlapping inferior alveolar canal, a panoramic radiograph shows following signs such as diversion of the inferior alveolar canal, darkening of the root, narrowing of the root and interruption of the white line all of which have been found to be significantly related to nerve injury.[4]

Because of their 2D images, panoramic radiographs provide limited information. The buccolingual relationship between the IAC and the lower third molar cannot be evaluated from panoramic radiographs. Furthermore, the presence or absence of cortication around the IAC and the detailed anatomy of the third molar may not be clearly evident with this method. The IAC could be detected without difficulty and located correctly in relation to the lower third molar in all of the CBCT scans. CBCT is more reliable in evaluating the number of mandibular third molar roots than panoramic radiography.[2] Neugebauer et al compared panoramic radiography and symmetric posteroanterior (PA) cephalometric radiography with CBCT imaging. They concluded that CBCT imaging improved the localization of third molars for presurgical planning.[2] Color coding of mandibular canal is now available with almost all CBCT softwares and third party software thereby allowing accurate visualization of the mandibular canal (Fig. 8.1).

Maxillary canines are the second most frequently impacted teeth after the third molars with prevalence from 1% to 3% (Figs 8.2A to E). The maxillary canine, in contrast to the third molar is located in a highly demanding area both functionally and esthetically. Most of the impactions are palatal (85%), whereas 15% are labial.[5]

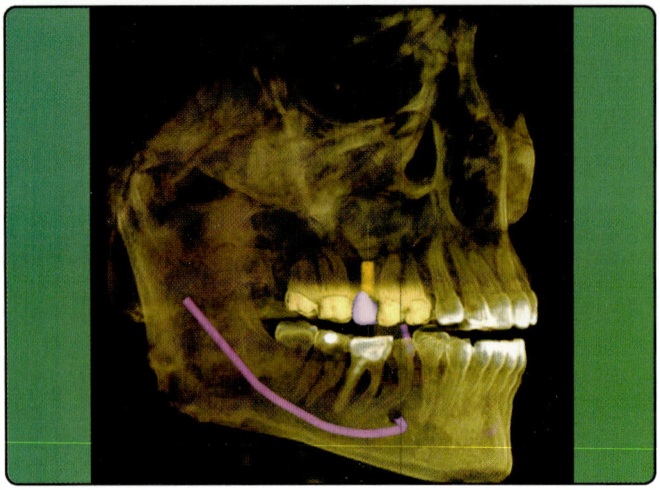

Figure 8.1: Color coding of the mandibular canal on cone beam computed tomography (Galileos, Sirona, Germany)

The CBCT allows description in all planes of space. 3D volumetric imaging might provide information for improved diagnosis and treatment plans, and ultimately result in more successful treatment outcomes and improved patient care.[5] In the maxilla, localization of impacted canines relative to the lateral and central incisors is central to their management. Information regarding the palatal orientation of an impacted canine and its proximity to the root of the lateral incisor is vital to allow for an effective and timely surgical intervention.[6] CBCT orthographic tomographic slices and panoramic reconstructions are superior to conventional panoramic radiographs in determining the location and orientation of an impacted tooth and its relationship to adjacent vital structures in the maxilla and the mandible. Supernumerary teeth are occasionally encountered by oral and maxillofacial clinicians (Figs 8.3A to C). Associated complications involve failure of adjacent teeth to erupt, displacement and crowding of the adjacent teeth, abnormal diastema, root resorption and even dentigerous cyst formation. Some cases of supernumeraries are asymptomatic and are only detected during radiographical examinations. Traditionally, radiographical information may be obtained by periapical, occlusal, panoramic or cephalometric radiographs. A single occlusal or periapical film gives the most detailed picture of the tooth in the incisor region, while the buccolingual position can be defined using the parallax technique namely, the horizontal tube shift technique. However, sometimes these cannot provide information about the 3D relationship of these supernumeraries to the associated teeth and neighboring structures, which is important in making decisions about treatment options (Table 8.1).[7]

Table 8.1: Cone beam computed tomography classification for supernumerary teeth[7]

Type of impaction	Position of supernumerary teeth
Type I	The supernumerary teeth were located palatal to the longitudinal axis of the neighboring normal incisor and inferior to its root apex
Type II	The supernumerary teeth were located superior and palatal to the neighboring incisors
Type III	The supernumerary teeth were located within the neck region of the normal arch (normally oriented) or transverse
Type IV	The supernumerary teeth were located superior to the root apex of the adjacent incisors (inverted or normally oriented) or obliquely across the root apex of the incisors
Type V	The supernumerary teeth were placed beyond the labial aspect of the root of the adjacent incisors
Type VI	The supernumerary teeth were placed palatal to the incisors, with the vertical position between that of type I or type II

The CBCT provides a picture of supernumeraries in three planes and in relation to neighboring structures at a significantly lower radiation dose compared with traditional spiral CT.

MAXILLOFACIAL TRAUMA

The aim of any imaging examination for maxillofacial injury is to demonstrate the positions of the anatomic elements, both hard and soft tissue, in three spatial planes. Single or combinations of conventional plain films are still advocated as the baseline radiographical screening assessment for the investigation of facial fractures. Their diagnostic accuracy is approximately 38% for orbital and maxillary fractures and they significantly underestimate the extent of blowout, Le Fort I and Le Fort II fractures. These deficiencies are related to the inherent 2D projection and superimposition of both hard and soft tissue structures onto the interpreted 'plane' of the radiograph. In patients with mandibular fractures, conventional skull radiography is usually supplemented with rotational panoramic radiography. It provides greater diagnostic accuracy in detecting mandibular fractures. However, an isolated modality is inadequate for the diagnosis of many fractures of the midfacial region. The importance of CT imaging in maxillofacial trauma cannot be overemphasized. CT has

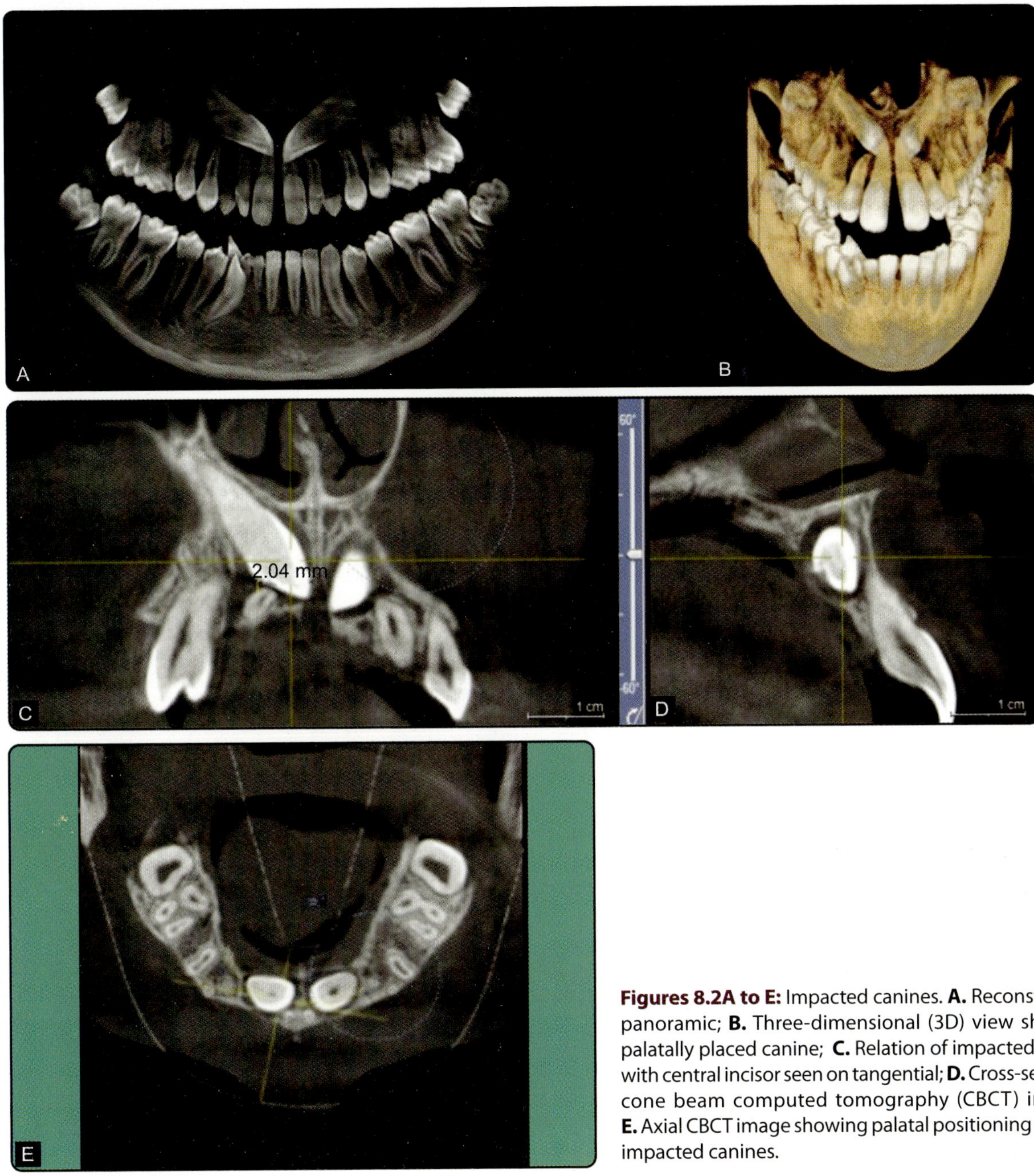

Figures 8.2A to E: Impacted canines. **A.** Reconstructed panoramic; **B.** Three-dimensional (3D) view showing palatally placed canine; **C.** Relation of impacted canine with central incisor seen on tangential; **D.** Cross-sectional cone beam computed tomography (CBCT) images; **E.** Axial CBCT image showing palatal positioning of both impacted canines.

become the imaging gold standard for assessing injuries to all regions of the maxillofacial skeleton. Although CT serves as the principal means of qualifying the clinical diagnosis of complex maxillofacial fractures, routine CT scanning may not be necessary in every case of facial trauma. There is, however, increasing support that CT findings are important determinants of surgical management. CT is the modality of choice for the evaluation of complex facial fractures, especially those involving the frontal sinus, nasoethmoidal region and the orbits.

Markowitz et al found coronal CT to be the most accurate method in the diagnosis of mandibular fractures followed by mandibular series and panoramic radiography. Interestingly they found axial CT detected significantly fewer angle fractures (60%) than standard radiographs (98%) and coronal CT (100%) and identified lack of fracture displacement was the single most important factor in missed fractures with all modalities. They recommended that in clinically stable and cooperative patients with mandibular trauma, panoramic radiography and coronal,

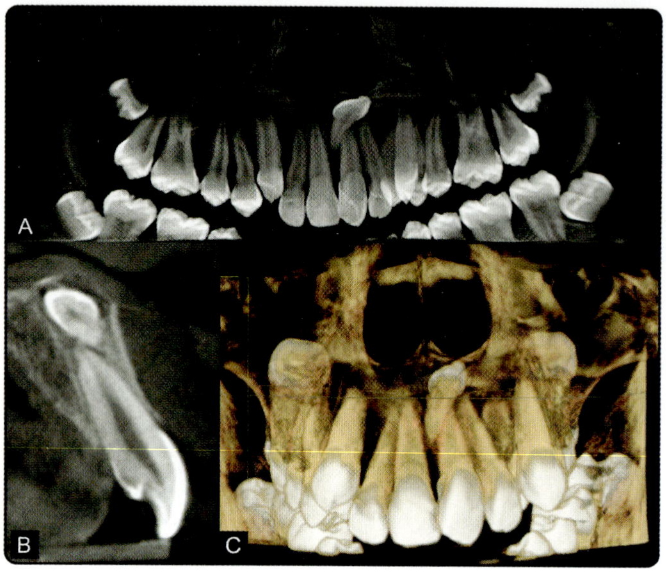

Figures 8.3A to C: Position of mesiodens accurately determined on cone beam computed tomography images. **A.** Reconstructed orthopantomogram (OPG); **B.** Cross-sectional image; **C.** Three-dimensional reconstruction.

not axial CT, is recommended to confirm clinical suspicions when the mandibular series is equivocal.

Perhaps the technology, with potentially the greatest impact on imaging in maxillofacial trauma in the current decade has been of CBCT. While the use of conventional CT has been limited because of cost, access, availability and dose considerations. Several CBCT systems are now available specifically for the maxillofacial region, providing increased opportunities for multiplanar reconstruction (MPR) and 3D imaging (Figs 8.4A and B). These units are particularly well-suited to imaging facial fractures.[8] Newer CBCT machines are now available in supine position also, thereby increasing its use in ambulatory patients suffering from maxillofacial trauma (Figs 8.5A and B).

With regard to the mandibular fractures, it has been stated that CBCT is superior to panoramic radiography as condylar and coronoid fractures and the anterior part of the mandible were more difficult to detect due to superimposition. Suspected mandibular fracture CBCT increases diagnostic certainty to 90.5%, even in situations when a change in treatment is not made (Figs 8.6A and B). Other possibilities for the use of CBCT exist for postoperative controls of the position of fragments and osteosynthesis plates and their relationship to endangered neighboring areas.[9]

CBCT IN MAXILLOFACIAL PATHOLOGIES

The CBCT diagnostic applications in the maxillofacial region include evaluating the presence of osseous defects in

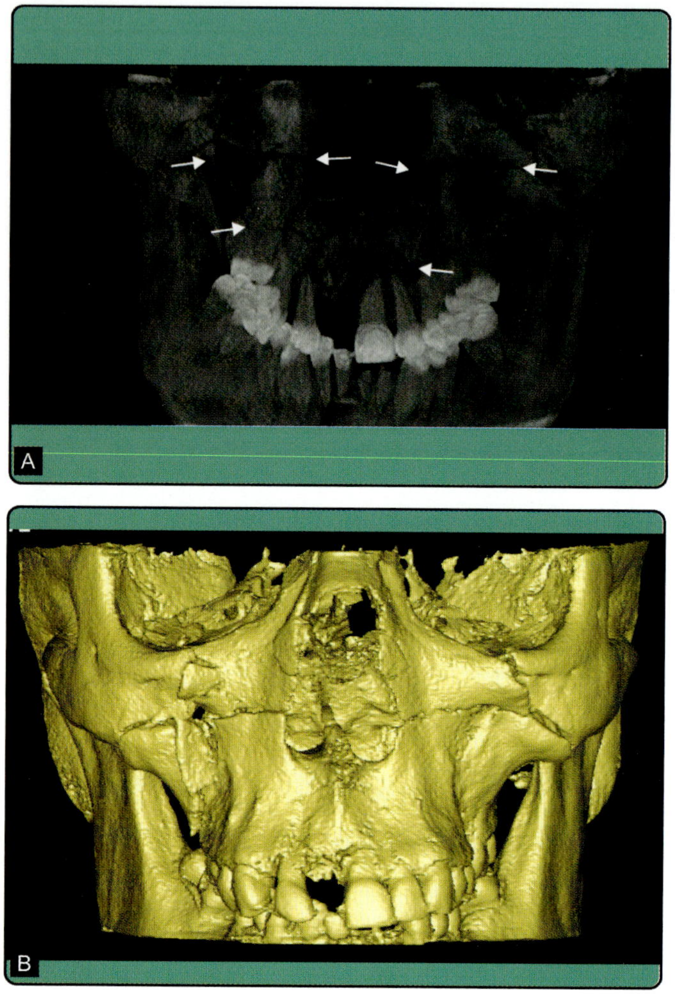

Figures 8.4A and B: Maxillofacial trauma. **A.** Posteroanterior image of zygomatic complex fracture; **B.** The three-dimensional (3D) reconstructed cone beam computed tomography.

the jaws, cysts, lesions, calcifications. CBCT is also playing an increasingly important role in the detection of 'incidental' pathology in patients referred for dental treatment. Since, most currently available CBCT systems acquire volumes that extend beyond the dentition and the surrounding alveolus, unsuspected lesions in the paranasal sinuses, parotic region, masticatory space, floor of the mouth and the hyoid region are frequently detected and reported. Evidently, the 3D nature of CBCT allows determination of the exact extension of the lesion in the affected region.[10]

Benign Lesions and Cysts

One of the primary benefits of CBCT is its capacity to display the scanned area in multiplanar orientation. In evaluating cysts or benign tumors, a single, intraoral radiograph may not fully record the entire dimensions of the lesion. Thus,

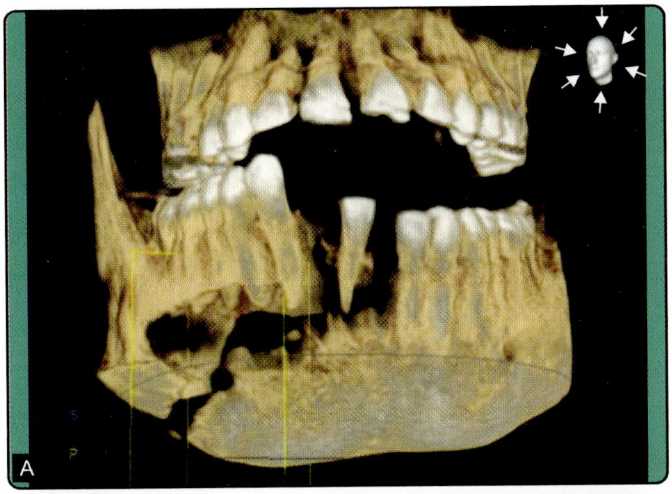

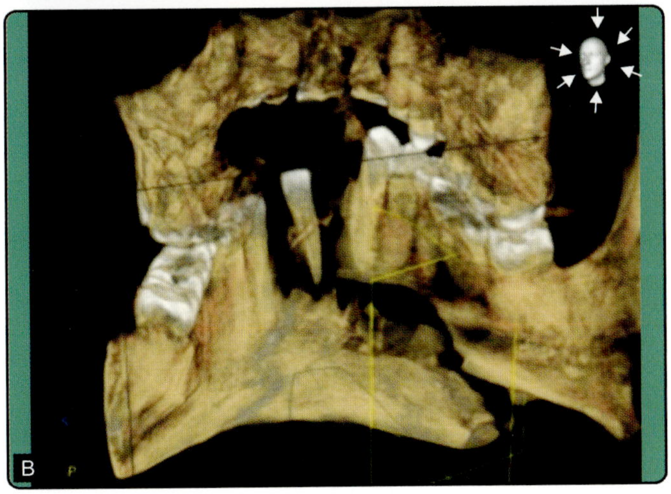

Figures 8.5A and B: The three-dimensional (3D) reconstructed cone beam computed tomography images (buccal/lingual view) of parasymphyseal fracture. **A.** Buccal view; **B.** Lingual view.

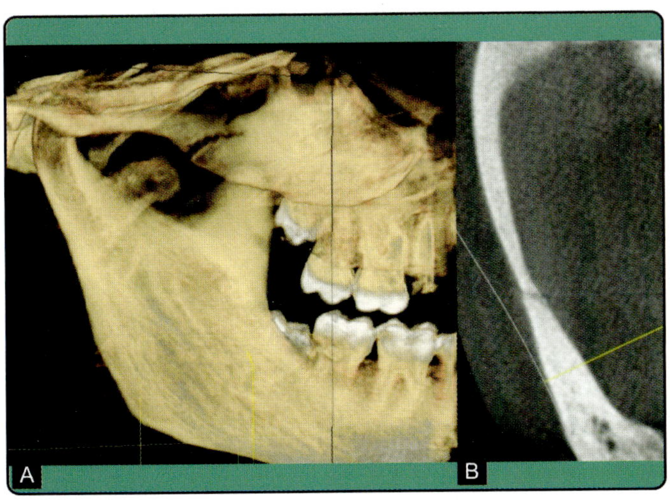

Figures 8.6A and B: Right zygomatic arch fracture. **A.** Three-dimensional (3D) reconstructed; **B.** Axial view.

multiple intraoral radiographs or a panoramical radiograph are often required. These multiple radiographs still show only the 2D of the lesion. Observation of the 3D, i.e. buccolingual extension of a lesion, requires additional radiographs obtained at 90° from the original view. In contrast, all 3D are recorded by multiplanar CBCT imaging. Such multiplanar views provide important information on the presence and extent of bone resorption, sclerosis of neighboring bone, cortical expansion and internal or external calcifications. 3D reconstructions are most useful for morphological analysis and spatial relationship of the neighboring structures for growth and developmental anomalies, gross tumor development or fracture displacement. Clinicians can depend on panoramic radiography for 2D information, if the margins of a cystic or benign lesion are well defined. If the margins are ill defined, CBCT is a better option for diagnosis. From a surgical perspective, this is especially important when evaluating potential areas of cortical perforation of aggressive benign cysts or tumors, e.g. odontogenic keratocysts (OKCs) or ameloblastomas (Figs 8.7 to 8.13A to E). Apart from presurgical evaluation of aggressive benign cysts or tumors, CBCT is also helpful in postsurgical follow-up of lesions that may have a high recurrence rate.[11]

Inflammatory Lesions

Acute inflammatory lesions cannot be diagnosed either on plain film radiography or on CBCT scan as 30% of calcified structures need to be affected before it is evident on radiograph. If an aggressive infection persists for 2 weeks or more, the primary finding on any radiographical examination is a lytic lesion with irregular

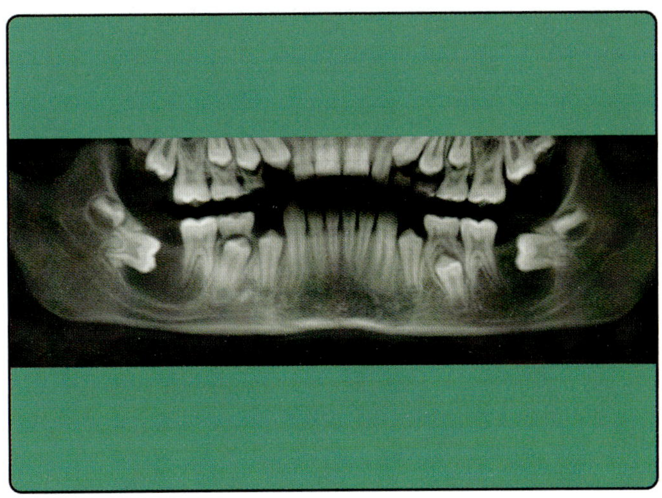

Figure 8.7: Panoramic cone beam computed tomography, showing second molars horizontally retained with pericoronal radiolucency lesions bilaterally.

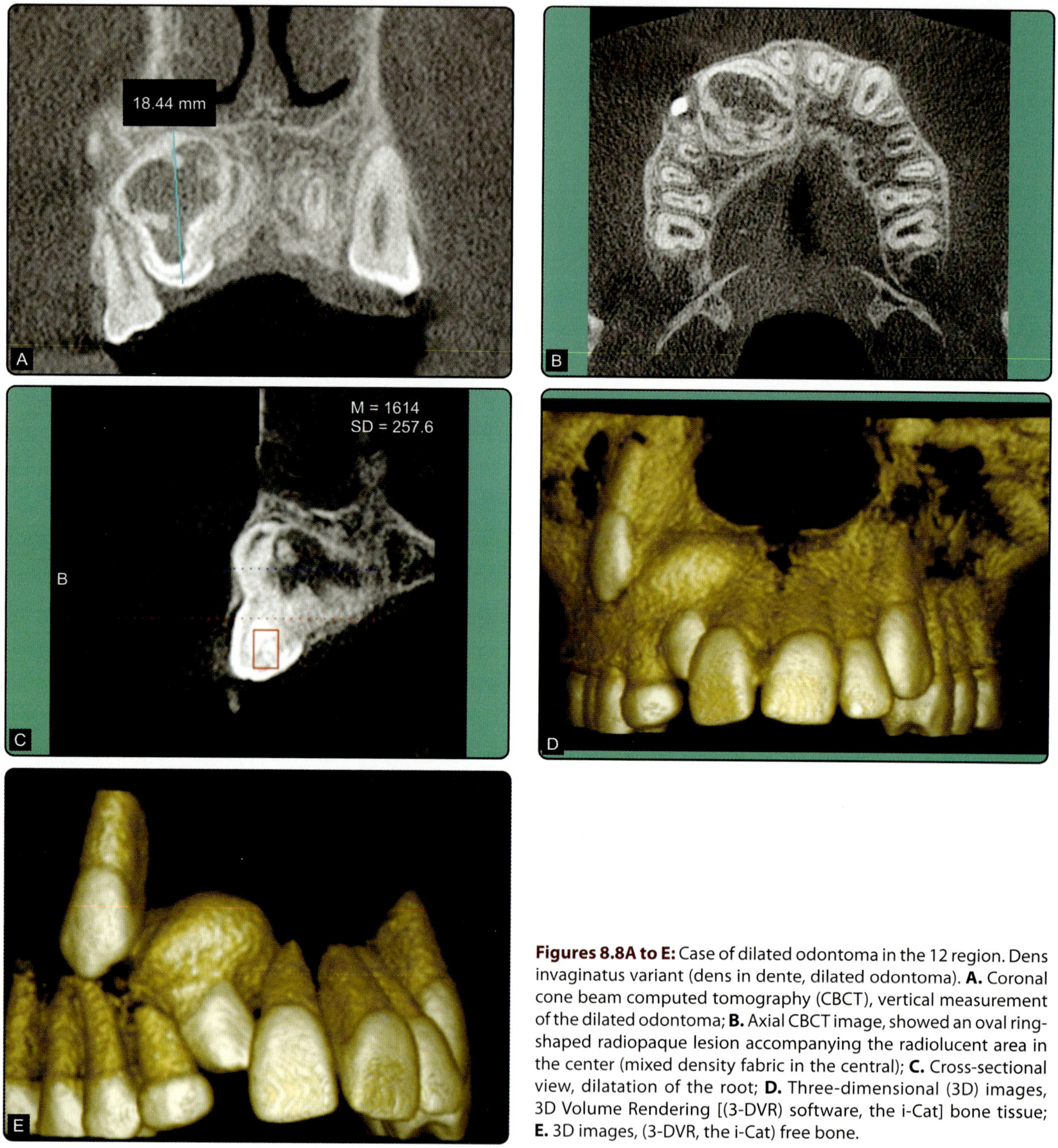

Figures 8.8A to E: Case of dilated odontoma in the 12 region. Dens invaginatus variant (dens in dente, dilated odontoma). **A.** Coronal cone beam computed tomography (CBCT), vertical measurement of the dilated odontoma; **B.** Axial CBCT image, showed an oval ring-shaped radiopaque lesion accompanying the radiolucent area in the center (mixed density fabric in the central); **C.** Cross-sectional view, dilatation of the root; **D.** Three-dimensional (3D) images, 3D Volume Rendering [(3-DVR) software, the i-Cat] bone tissue; **E.** 3D images, (3-DVR, the i-Cat) free bone.

margins. If the infection is chronic or moderate to low grade, the bone appears to be of mixed density. As a defense mechanism, the body walls the infection off by depositing layers of periosteal bone. Additionally, the margin of a chronic infection is often sclerotic with periosteal reaction, which can be adequately viewed

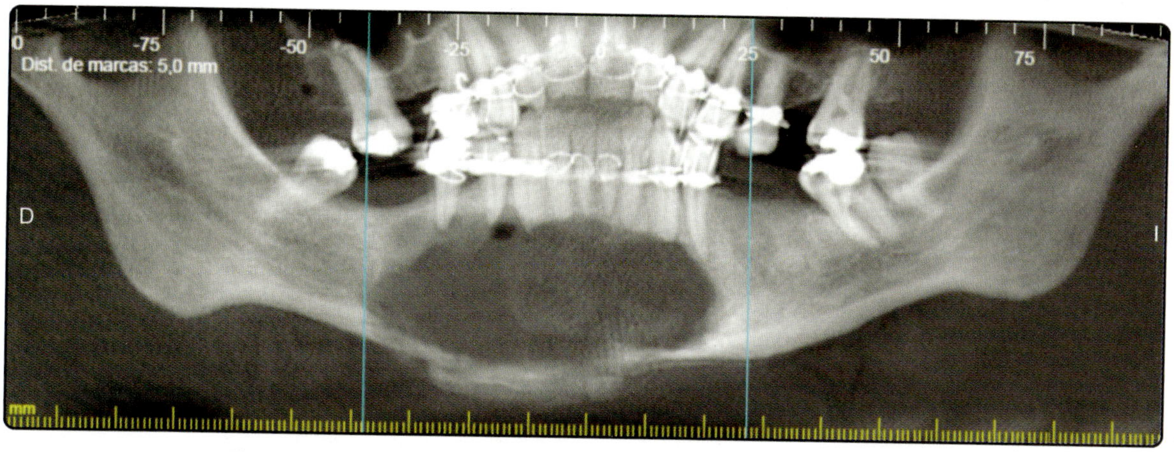

Figure 8.9: Central giant cell granuloma, after treatment with curettage

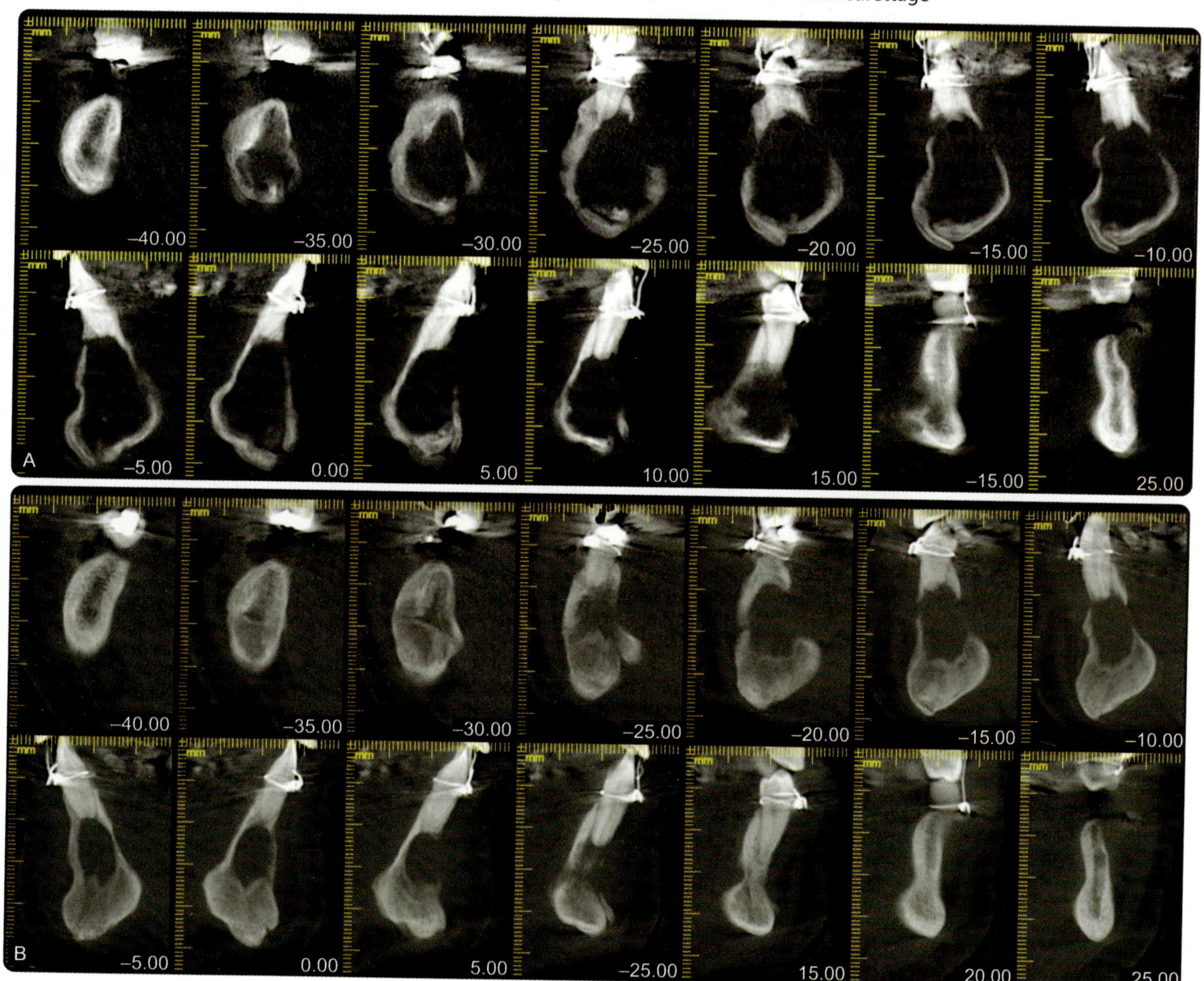

Figures 8.10A and B: Central giant cell granuloma after treatment with curettage. **A.** Panoramic and cross section in the anterior of the mandible (cuts every 5 mm), control 3 months after surgery; **B.** Cross section in the anterior of the mandible (cuts every 5 mm), control 7 months after surgery.

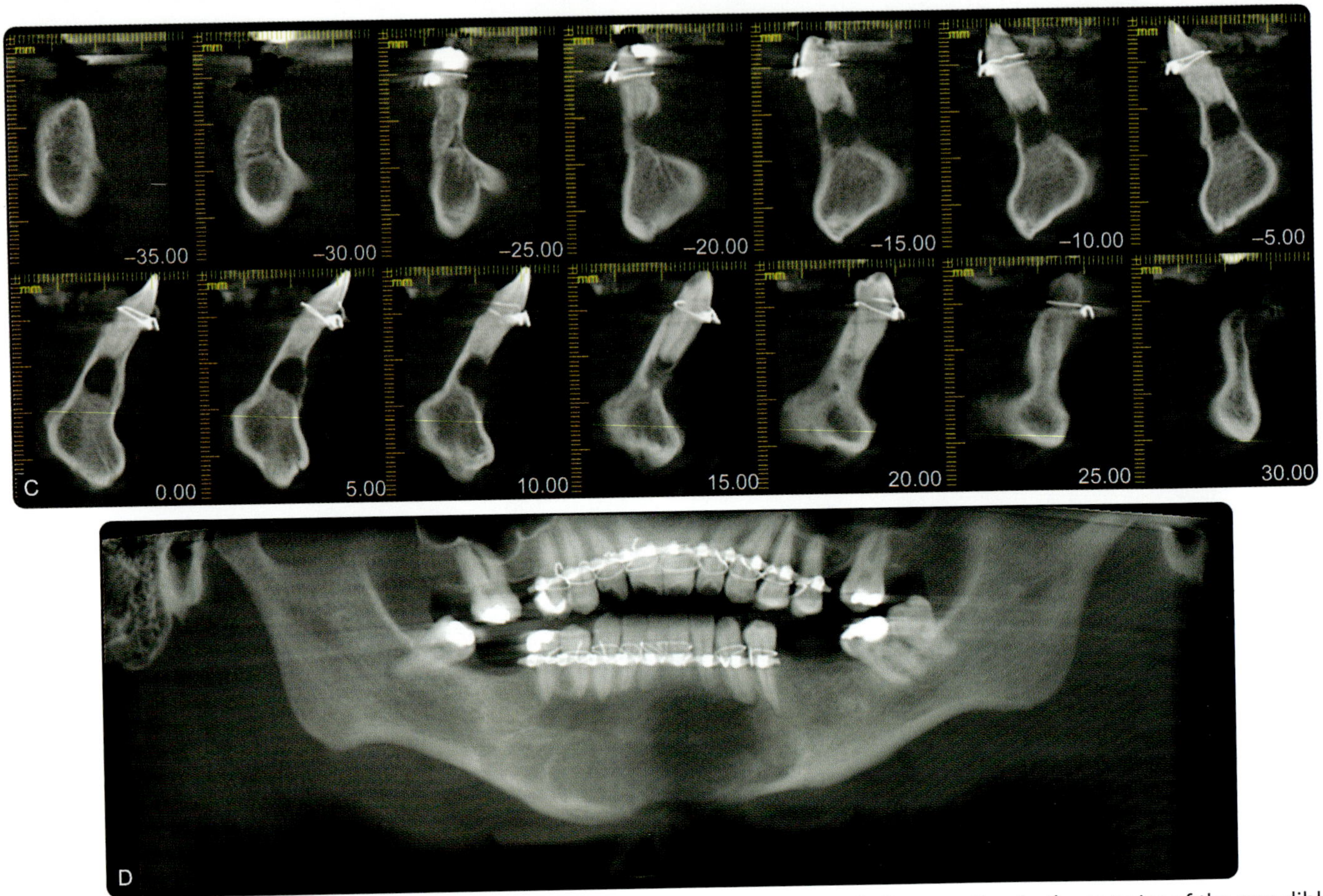

Figures 8.10C and D: Central giant cell granuloma after treatment with curettage; **C.** Cross section in the anterior of the mandible (cuts every 5 mm), control—1 year 4 months after surgery; **D.** Panoramic cone beam computed tomography, control—1 year 4 months after surgery.

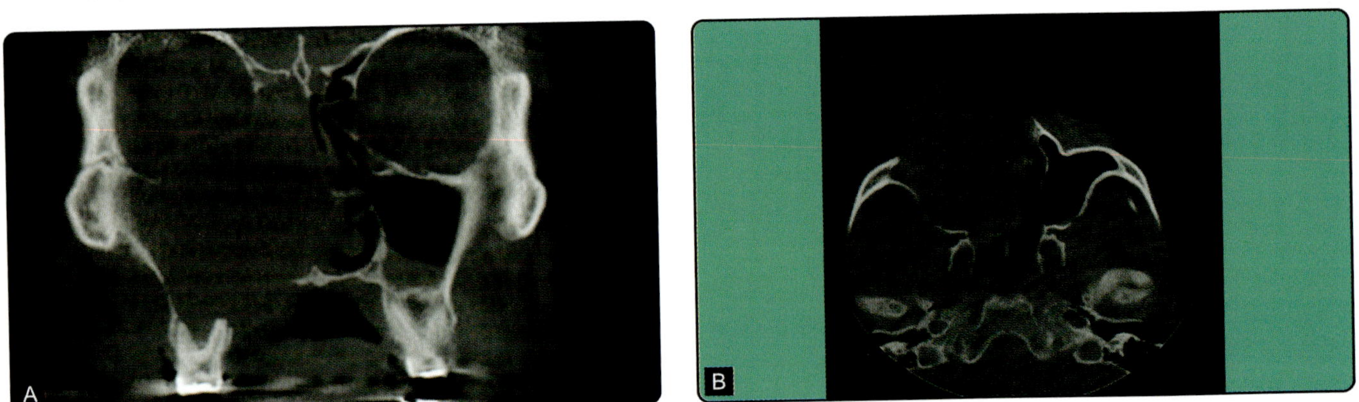

Figures 8.11A and B: Coronal and axial cone beam computed tomography, demonstrating the large tumor (central giant cell tumor) mass involving the entire right maxilla, and maxillary and ethmoid sinuses and compressing nose. **A.** Coronal view; **B.** Axial view.

on plain film radiographs (Figs 8.14A to E). With CBCT images, diagnosing new periosteal bone formation resulting from osteomyelitis is easier since the thin bone layer can be viewed by changing image orientation and adjusting density and contrast. From a surgical perspective, when compared with plain film, CBCT is better able to manifest small bony sequestra associated with osteomyelitis, which requires surgical debridement.[11]

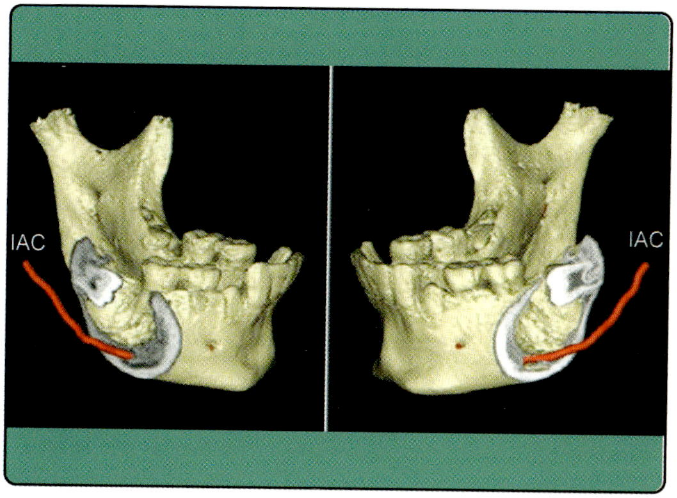

Figure 8.12: The three-dimensional (3D) reconstruction showing bilateral dentigerous cyst involving mandibular canal (3D SimPlant materialize) (IAC, inferior alveolar canal).

Foreign Body Detection

Compared to CBCT images, multiple detector computed tomography (MDCT) images have superior soft-tissue resolution. In the maxillofacial area, the soft-tissue information on a MDCT scan can be degraded by artifacts arising from metal restorations. Extensive bridgework can make a MDCT scan virtually nondiagnostic. Such artifacts from metal objects are lower on CBCT images. Therefore, a CBCT is a better imaging modality to assess metal fragments in the face, such as fragments embedded from a gunshot, automobile or industrial accidents and for localizing retained broken dental needles.[11]

Soft-tissue Calcifications

Although CBCT images have low-contrast (soft tissue) resolution, they can be better than MDCT in depicting soft-tissue calcifications such as carotid atherosclerosis. Other calcifications such as tonsilloliths and sialoliths are adequately viewed on CBCT images (Figs 8.15A and B). Small calcifications, which can be important diagnostic clues for some types of cysts and tumors, e.g. calcifying epithelial odontogenic tumor (CEOT) or Pindborg tumor calcifying odontogenic cyst (COC) or Gorlin cyst are easier to identify on a CBCT scan than panoramic or intraoral radiographs.[11]

CBCT IN ORAL CANCER AND OSTERADIONECROSIS

Oral squamous cell carcinomas (OSCC) may be adjacent or fixed to the mandible/maxilla. The treatment of choice for these carcinomas is wide excision of the tumor in the soft tissue 'en bloc' with the involved bone and postoperative radiotherapy depending on the final histopathology results. The preoperative extent of mandibular bone involvement is often difficult to assess because no single imaging method is able to predict mandibular invasion

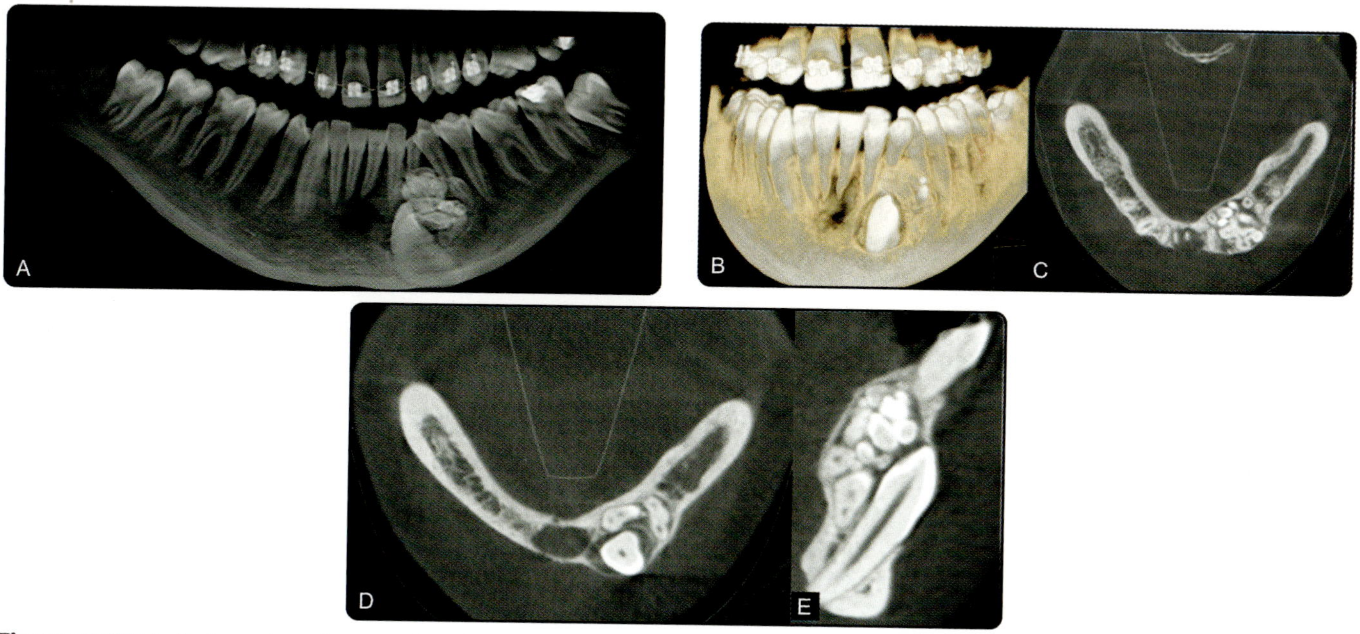

Figures 8.13A to E: Complex odontoma interfering with eruption of canine clearly viewed on cone beam computed tomography images. **A.** Reconstructed orthopantomogram (OPG); **B.** Three-dimensional reconstruction; **C** and **D.** Axial view; **E.** Cross-sectional view.

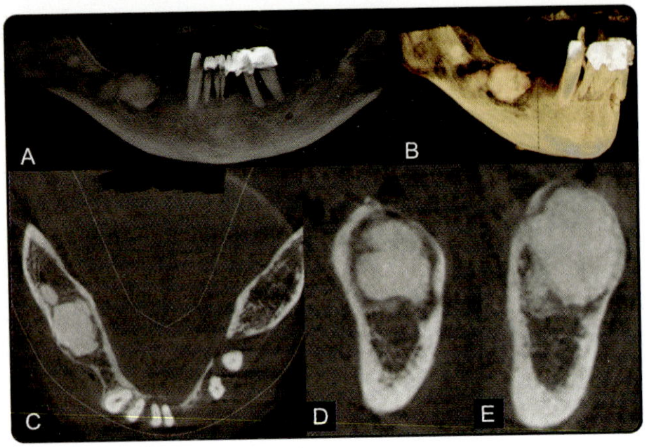

Figures 8.14A to E: Focal sclerosing osteomyelitis clearly depicted on cone beam computed tomography images. **A.** Reconstructed orthopantomogram (OPG); **B.** Three-dimensional reconstruction; **C.** Axial view; **D** and **E.** Cross-sectional view.

and the extent of invasion 100% reliably. CBCT seems of great value for the prediction of mandibular invasion by OSCC, adjacent to or fixed to the mandible. Initial study on CBCT used for mandibular invasion by OSCC revealed that CBCT was significantly superior to panoramic radiography in evaluating mandibular invasion by lower gingival carcinoma.[12] Although CBCT may predict the presence or absence of mandibular invasion, the goal is to depict the extent of mandibular invasion accurately (Figs 8.16A and B). CBCT and MSCT tend to underestimate and MRI tends to overestimate the extent of mandibular invasion. Bone single-photon emission computerized tomography (SPECT) also overestimates the extent as increased tracer uptake extends beyond the area of mandibular invasion and the gamma camera has limited spatial resolution. CBCT has many advantages over MSCT. The major advantages include the upright position of the patient in CBCT compared with the supine position in MSCT. This might offer more accurate information because the soft tissues do not tend to collapse dorsally. CBCT involves less radiation than MSCT and could therefore be used in a wider range of patients. The radiation dose for OSCC imaging using CBCT is four times higher than panoramic radiography. At present, dynamic contrast-enhanced (DCE) MRI seems a promising imaging technique for the delineation of mandibular invasion. Small lesions on cortical bone such as mucoepidermoid carcinoma on the hard palate are difficult to diagnose using panoramic or occlusal radiographs. If clinical examination suggests such a lesion, a small field of view CBCT scan can reveal the extent of the tumor.[11]

Bisphosphonate-associated osteonecrosis of the jaws (BONJ) is a well-defined complication of bisphosphonate therapy. Although the prevalence is much greater in cancer patients treated with high-dose intravenous (IV) formulations, BONJ has also been reported in patients taking oral bisphosphonates for management of osteoporosis. The condition is characterized by exposed non-vital maxillary or mandibular bone that may be associated with localized soft tissue infection, pain, swelling, purulent discharge, paresthesia, extraoral fistula formation and pathologic fracture. The two most widely used and consistently reported imaging modalities in reports of BONJ are panoramic tomography and CT. Fragmentation and sequestrum formation can be associated with pain and may require surgical intervention; CBCT is clearly superior in detecting this feature.

Temporomandibular Joint Imaging

The temporomandibular joint (TMJ) is a complex entity with hard- and soft-tissue components. TMJ disorders (TMDs) are common, but widely variable. MRI has sustained its position as the gold standard imaging modality for diagnosing TMDs since it provides excellent visibility of the disk and the associated joint muscles. Nonetheless,

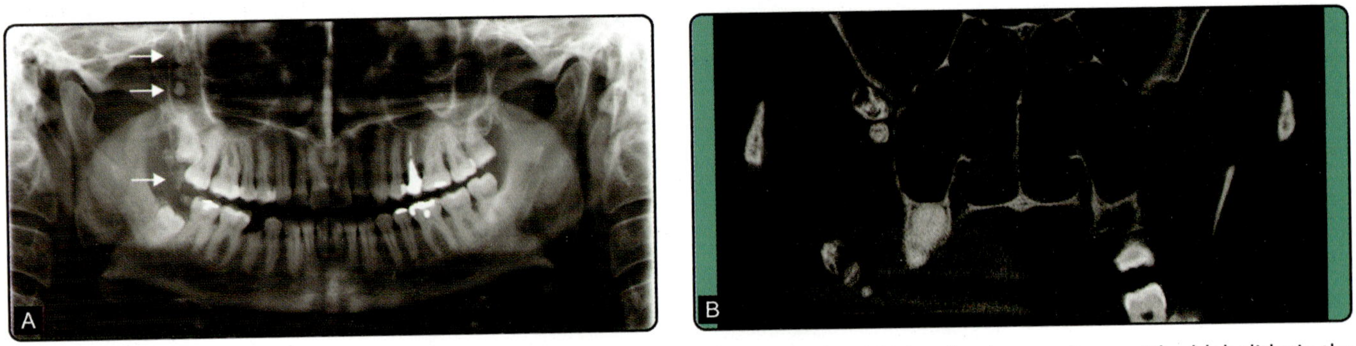

Figures 8.15A and B: Panoramic and coronal cone beam computed tomography (CBCT) showing hemangioma with phleboliths in the infratemporal space. **A.** Panoramic radiograph showing radiopacities overspray posterior maxillary sinus, pterygoid fossa and area behind the molars (arrows indicated); **B.** The CBCT coronal section, showing in the right infratemporal space several round calcified foci.

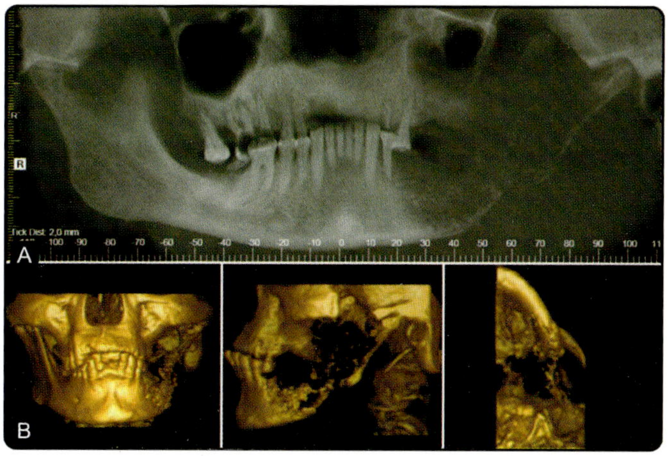

Figures 8.16A and B: Carcinoma in jaw bone ('carcinoma epidermoide'). **A.** Panoramic cone beam computed tomography showing posterior mandibular extensive bone destruction; **B.** Three-dimensional (3D) volume rendering by i-Cat software.

most TMJ examinations start with a panoramical radiography to visualize any gross changes in the condylar head and temporal components. However, panoramical radiography has a low diagnostic accuracy in detecting TMDs so a negative indicator on a panoramical radiography does not exclude the presence of osseous defect. Conventional radiography has some limitations. The morphology of the central and medial parts of TMJ cannot be investigated in these radiographs because of the superimpositions. Only the angle of the most lateral posterior slope of the eminence is visible in the conventional radiography. No slices can be made with the conventional films, so these examinations do not depict an accurate representation of articular eminence morphology. Overall, modalities, which are imaging only one slice such as conventional tomography or those modalities, which project no slices such as conventional films cannot precisely assess the inclination of the articular eminence. Hintze et al noted accurate assessment of joint morphology is very difficult on panoramic radiographs due to distortion of the joints. The panoramic radiography only represents the most lateral part of the articular eminence. Accurate measurements on panoramical radiography are affected by several factors such as projection geometry, patient positioning, focal plane shape and magnification factors.[13]

The CBCT parasagittal and coronal slices show crisp, clear images of the condylar head and the glenoid fossa. CBCT is more accurate than panoramic radiography and conventional tomography for detecting TMDs thereby influencing the treatment plan. CT provides optimal imaging of the osseous components of the TMJ with 87.5%–96% accuracy in detecting degenerative arthritis.[14]

Remodeling

Remodeling is a physiological process that aims to adapt the structure of TMJ to the mechanical forces applied to the joint. Excessive forces may cause alteration of the shape of the condyle and articular eminence. This adaptive response may result in a flattening of curved joint surfaces, increased bone density (sclerosis) and absence of destruction or degeneration of articular soft tissue. These findings are easily diagnosed on CBCT scans.[11]

Osteoarthritis

Degenerative arthritis or osteoarthritis is an age-related disorder and the most common pathological condition of the TMJ. Osteoarthritic bony changes include irregular cortical outlines, erosions, osteophyte formation, subchondral cyst formation, resorption of the condylar head and reduced joint space. These changes are most commonly seen on the condyle, but may also involve the mandibular fossa or articular eminence. A joint with osteoarthritic changes may also demonstrate flattening or sclerosis. CBCT is a valuable imaging technique for the diagnosis of degenerative changes of the TMJ. CBCT images also provide superior reliability and greater accuracy than corrected angle linear tomography and TMJ panoramical projections in the detection of condylar cortical erosion.[11]

Inflammatory Arthritis

A general classification of arthritis divides the diseases into inflammatory, degenerative, infectious, metabolic and traumatic categories. When an inflammatory disorder of the TMJ is suspected, CBCT is recommended for evaluation of subtle abnormalities. Both joints should be imaged for comparison. Cortical erosions most often involve the articular eminence and the anterior aspect of the condylar head. CBCT images also show subchondral sclerosis, flattening of articulating surfaces, subchondral cysts and osteophyte formation.[11]

Internal Derangement

Internal derangement of the TMJ is defined as an abnormal positional relationship of the disk relative to the mandibular condyle and articular eminence. Clinically, the derangement may be indicated by clicking in the affected joint or by a restricted opening. Clicking in the TMJ associated with the internal derangement is usually due to the disk displacement being reduced during the opening movement, but a derangement that does not reduce and is associated with restricted opening is characterized as close locked. The disk cannot be visualized with CBCT. If clinically indicated, MRI is the method of choice to provide definitive diagnostic information for the TMJ soft-tissue components. The concentric, posterior or lateral localization of the condyle within the joint space in closed position should be evaluated on the CBCT images.[11]

Ankylosis

Ankylosis is a fibrous or bony union between joint components and can be caused by trauma, rheumatoid arthritis or infection. Conventional images may reveal little useful information other than a limited amount of condylar translation. A CBCT examination is recommended, if ankylosis is clinically suspected as it provides superior visualization of the osseous components. In fibrous ankylosis, the articulating surfaces are usually irregular because of erosions and joint space is narrow. In bony ankylosis, no joint space at least in parts of the joint is visible. Secondary degenerative changes are common.[11]

In the study conducted by Hilgers et al the size of the condyle (height, width and length) and intercondylar, TMJ—mandible and mandibular spatial relationships were investigated with linear measurement with the iCAT (Xoran Technologies, Ann Arbor, Michigan; Imaging Sciences International, Hatfield, Pennsylvania) CBCT scanner. The linear measurements were same as on the dry skull. ProMax 3D CBCT images could accurately depict the TMJ space.[15] CBCT can provide submillimeter spatial resolution images with shorter scanning time, lower radiation dose and being more cost-effective than helical CT imaging.[13] A CBCT examination is also recommended before image-guided puncture operation of the superior compartment of the joint space.

Cleft Lip and Palate

Among congenital malformations, facial, cleft lip and palate anomalies are considered to be the most frequent representing the second most observed genetic defect in the population and constituting a serious dental, medical and social problem with a significant impact on esthetics, function and the affected patients' quality of life.

In cleft lip and palate patients, information regarding the number and orientation of teeth, dental and skeletal age and the amount and quality of available bone in the cleft region are considered vital for the clinical management of such cases. Alveolar bone graft is an essential procedure in the overall management of patients with cleft bone defect. It provides stability of the upper dental arch, gives bone support for the teeth adjacent to the cleft area, supports the lip and the nose, restores facial asymmetry, closes the residual oronasal fistula and provides bone support for dental implants in prosthetic rehabilitation.[16]

Panoramical radiography is often used to investigate the incidence and number of missing teeth and to determine dental and skeletal age in cleft lip and palate patients. However, the amount and quality of available bone cannot be accurately assessed on a panoramic radiograph. Therefore, medical CT (MSCT) is typically used to quantify the amount of bone present, but the young age of cleft patients makes the routine use of MSCT problematic due to the relatively high-radiation dose involved. CBCT is rapidly replacing medical CT for this task since it provides excellent 3D visualization of the palate at the premaxilla region at a lower patient dose. CBCT is used to determine dental age and when a large scan field of view (FOV) selection is present, 3D reconstructions of the cervical vertebra can be made and employed to determine skeletal age. Additionally, CBCT has been used to show any deformities in the piriform margin in the nasal platform and the anteroposterior depression of the nasal alar base. 3D CBCT reconstructions of the skin surface of the face and nose for cleft lip assessment are also possible (Figs A to E 8.17). The use of CT using 3D protocols provided an excellent visualization of the bone architecture and this is considered to be a valuable tool in the evaluation of craniofacial deformities in patients with congenital malformations such as cleft palate and alveolar ridge. The accurate and reliable diagnosis of the size and extent of bone defects caused by oral clefts is important not only in the treatment planning but also to establish the donor area and the volume of bone graft used in the therapeutic process for these patients. It is reported that MSCT and CBCT are reliable techniques in the volumetric assessment of bone defects in alveolar

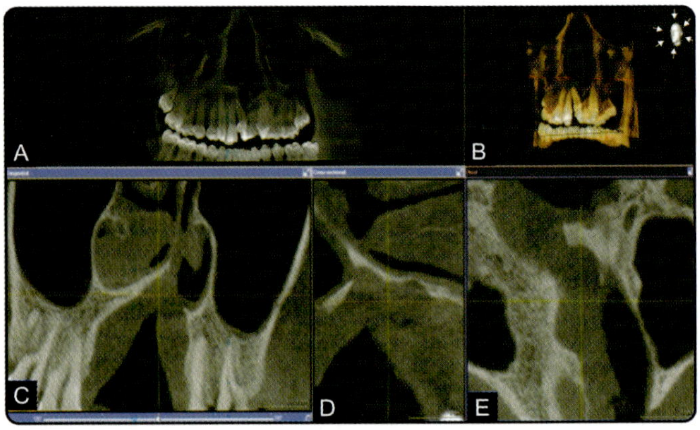

Figures 8.17A to E: Cone beam computed tomography images showing extend of cleft defect on left side (Orthophos XG 3D, Sirona, Germany). **A.** Reconstructed panoramic view; **B.** Three-dimensional (3D) view; **C.** Tangential view; **D.** Cross-sectional view; **E.** Axial view.

and palatal regions except for the greater radiation dose in case of MSCT.

During recent years, stereophotogrammetry has evolved. With the introduction of systems such as the 3dMDfaceTM System (3dMD LLC, Atlanta, United States of America), Di3DTM (Dimensional Imaging, Glasgow, United Kingdom) and 3D Sensoren FaceSCAN3D (3D-Shape GmbH, Erlangen, Germany), the applicability of 3D photographs in daily practice has become reality. 3D stereophotogrammetry is safe, noninvasive and able to capture superior quality 'external surface' photographs in less than 2 ms (Fig. 8.18). These characteristics make it ideal to collect the 3D data of faces, even in children or babies. After processing the data, an accurate digital model of the patient's face is created that can be used immediately in a clinical setting. 3D stereophotogrammetry is a sensitive, quick and non-invasive method for capturing and evaluating the changes of the nose after rhinoplasty in cleft lip or cleft palate patients. Disadvantages of the system are the need for carefully controlled lighting conditions and the use of four to six high-resolution cameras, making it a relatively non-portable system, while the cost of the setup can reach $50,000 or more.[17]

CBCT IN EARS, NOSE AND THROAT

Currently, a few CBCT manufacturers are marketing their units to otorhinolaryngologists as an efficient in office imaging tool. The benefit of using a CBCT in an ears, nose and throat (ENT) office is to identify less-complicated disease conditions quickly, cheaply and with lower radiation dose compared to a MDCT examination. In many situations, an ENT specialist obtains adequate information on a CBCT scan to render a diagnosis. CBCT scans are also used to select cases that need further examinations. For a dentist, identifying the condition of the maxillary sinuses is important for implant planning, endodontic therapy and also to rule out sinus disease as a cause for orofacial pain. Sinusitis, a common inflammatory disease involving the maxillofacial skeleton, is often of odontogenic origin. In some cases with sinusitis, endodontic therapy of the offending tooth may fail, requiring surgical intervention.

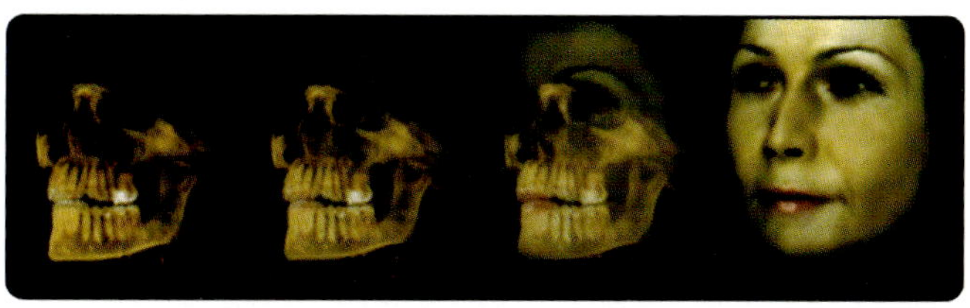

Figure 8.18: Virtual facial reconstruction with face scanner (Galileos, Sirona, Germany)

If sinusitis originates from the first maxillary molar, the periapical lesion is associated with the palatal root in 53% of cases. If the causative tooth is a second molar, a periapical lesion of the mesiobuccal root causes the highest occurrence (60%). CBCT not only provides diagnostic information of the status of extension of periapical lesions into the maxillary sinuses but also provides reliable information on the septa of the sinus and presence of exostoses. This is a useful presurgical information when planning sinus floor augmentation in preparation for implant placement. For the purpose of diagnosing sinus disease, altering the scan time is not required. A long acquisition time may provide better image quality and less noise compared to a short scan, but the images appear to have similar diagnostic value.

Studies show that Waters' sinus views are inadequate in detecting maxillary sinus opacification and 'very poor' in detecting masses in the ethmoid, frontal and sphenoid sinuses. These studies recommend the use of a low-dose and high-resolution multiplanar examination to evaluate the sinuses. CBCT images are also helpful in identifying mucus retention phenomena, antral polyps, sinonasal polyposis and malignant tumors of the sinuses. In addition, a dentist should consider a CBCT scan if there is a suspicion of oroantral fistula formation or if an implant is displaced into the sinus. Limitation of CBCT is its poor resolution of soft tissues. Sinus masses can be composed of different types of soft tissues with or without fluid accumulation (Figs 8.19 and 8.20).

In addition, the fluid may be a thin watery secretion, blood or a purulent mixture. On a CBCT scan, a mass in the sinus usually has a uniform density. Therefore, differentiation of the density into a fluid or soft-tissue mass is often not reliable. CBCT data can be relied on for the size and margin of the sinus mass, status of the sinus wall and blockage of the ostium. Some software allows accurate measurement of the air space. Fungal sinusitis often accumulates calcified materials. On a CBCT scan, these calcified materials can be easily differentiated from the soft-tissue component of the sinusitis.[11]

CBCT IN SALIVARY GLAND DISEASES

Major salivary glands can present a variety of lesions, which can appear clinically as a lateral facial swelling or diffuse glandular enlargement accompanied by symptoms of obstruction or inflammation. Salivary gland disorders commonly caused due to sialolith, bacterial or viral infections, autoimmune disorders like Sjögren's syndrome, benign and malignant salivary gland diseases. Radiographical examination is essential in diagnosing the lesions and useful for planning further management, whether surgery or alternatives. Plain radiography, sialography, CT, CBCT, ultrasonography (US), MRI and nuclear scintigraphy/positron emission tomography (PET) all play roles in the diagnosis of salivary gland lesions.[18] Sialography is the mainstay of salivary gland disease diagnosis.

Despite several limitations of sialography, it remains widely used for the diagnosis of salivary gland diseases, which affect the ductal system; in addition, it provides the ability to assess the suitability for interventional procedures and radiolucent stones. Although CT and US have been used, they have shown to be of limited value in visualizing the ductal system. However, a reliable technique that generates reproducible results similar to those of sialography has yet to emerge.[19]

The CBCT has recently become widespread in maxillofacial radiology due to its high-resolution and low-radiation dose. It offers improvement in demonstration of the ductal system over conventional sialography. CBCT recently has shown its potential in diagnosing salivary gland disorders like stenosis, ductal evagination, dilatation, stones or filling defects and space occupying lesions (Figs 8.21A to D, to 8.25A to D).[18]

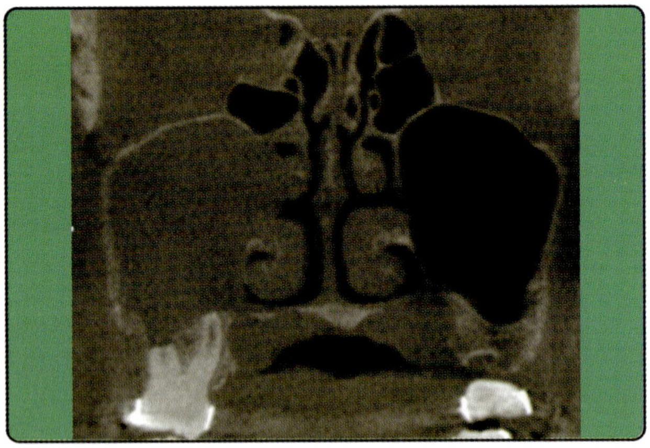

Figure 8.19: Left odontogenic sinusitis secondary to molar infection

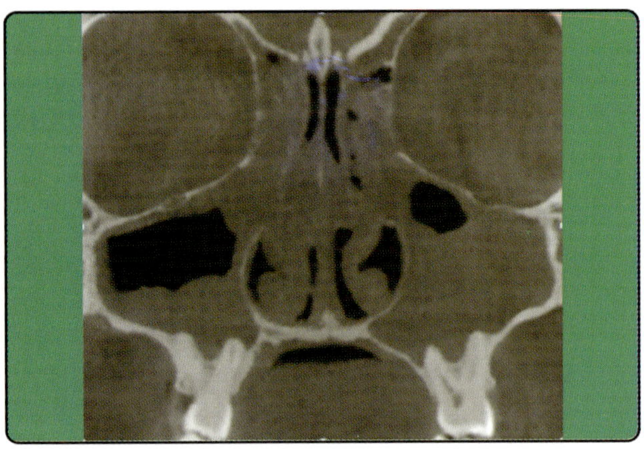

Figure 8.20: Coronal view on cone beam computed tomography showing pan sinusitis

Conventional sialography uses panoramic, occlusal and posteroanterior radiographs, which provide appropriate views for examining the major salivary glands. Moreover, recently it has been observed that CBCT sialography easily surpasses the shortcomings of the conventional sialography with predictable and precise diagnosis. Due to the isotropic voxels, the images of the anatomic structures can be reconstructed clearly and accurately in any plane in CBCT. Li et al studied the diagnosis of simple bone cysts by CBCT sialography. They noted that the sialography technique could be improved by the combination of sialography and CBCT, especially by 3D formatting.[20] Regarding the effective doses from CBCT examinations centered on the parotid and submandibular glands, Jadu et al concluded that they were similar to those calculated for plain radiography for sialography when 15 cm field of view (FOV) was chosen in combination with exposure conditions of 80 kVp and 10 mA.[21]

They compared 2D sialography with CBCT sialography and found that CBCT sialography may be better than plain film sialography in visualizing the delicate structures of the parotid and submandibular salivary glands, identifying sialoliths and single ductal strictures, as well as differentiating normal salivary glands from those with secondary inflammatory changes. In conclusion, in cases that have obstructive salivary gland diseases, it would be

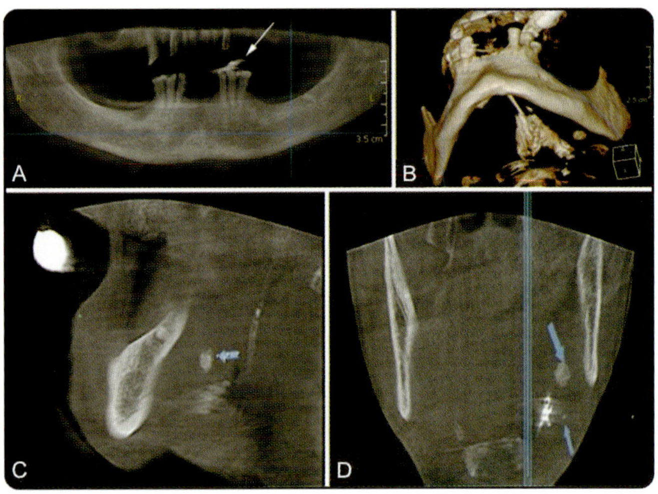

Figures 8.21A to D: Panoramical view. **A.** Three-dimensional (3D) reconstruction; **B.** Sagittal; **C.** Coronal; **D.** Images of cone beam computed tomography with large and small stones in the submandibular gland (arrows).

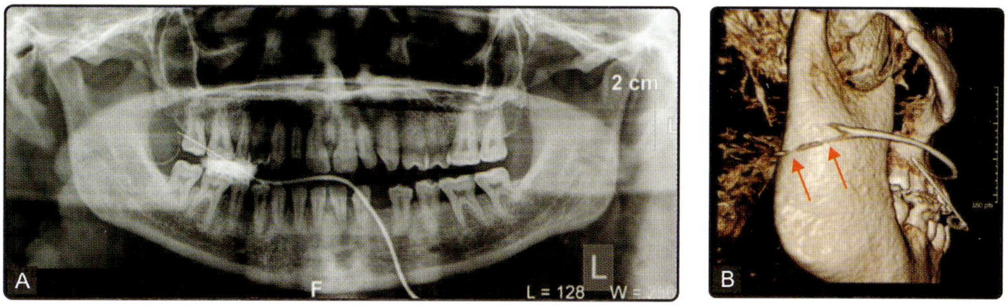

Figures 8.22A and B: Sialography. **A.** Panoramic sialogram shows stenosis of the right Stensen's duct; **B.** Cone beam computed tomography sialography three-dimensional (3D) reconstruction show stenosis with areas of strictures through the glandular ductules (arrows).

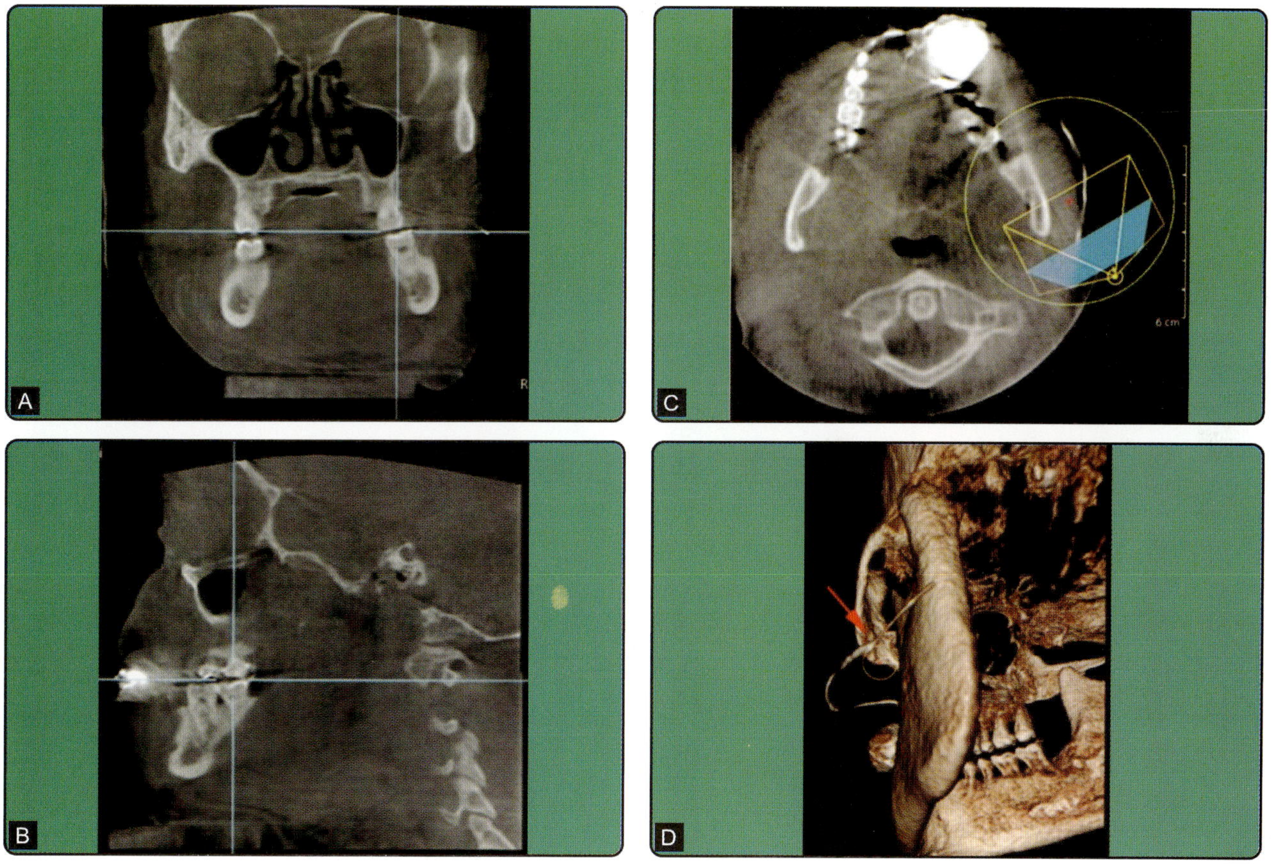

Figures 8.23A to D: Coronal view. **A.** Sagittal; **B.** Axial; **C.** Three-dimensional (3D) reconstruction; **D.** image showing multiple stenoses in Stensen's duct (arrow).

that have obstructive salivary gland diseases, it would be advisable to perform CBCT sialography as the modality of choice in demonstrating the ductal system of the gland and as an alternative to conventional sialography.

CONCLUSION

The CBCT is a fantastic imaging modality for diagnosis and treatment planning of maxillofacial pathologies.

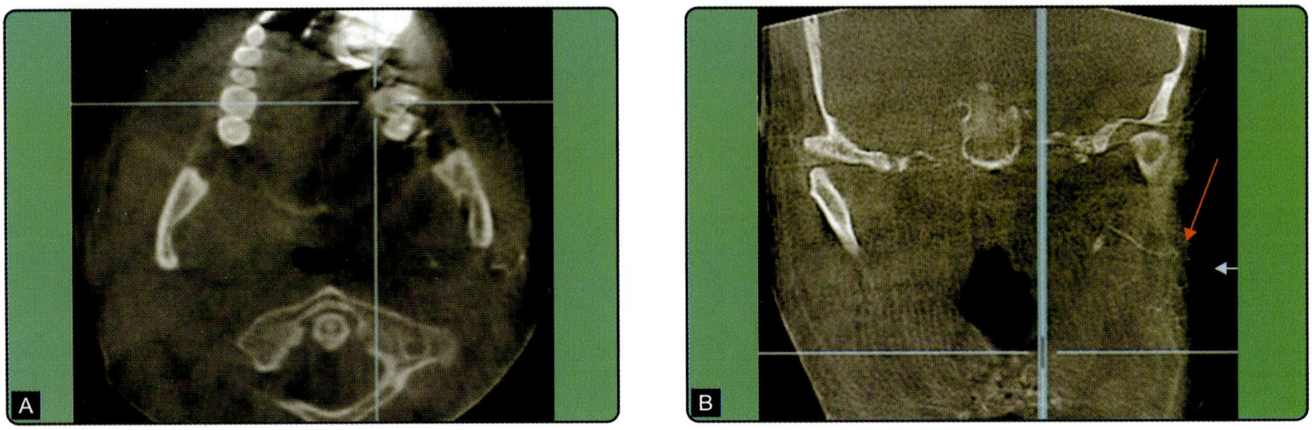

Figures 8.24A and B: Axial cut. **A.** Coronal cut; **B**. Cut of cone beam computed tomography sialography showing stenosis of the ductules with punctuated appearance of the gland (arrow).

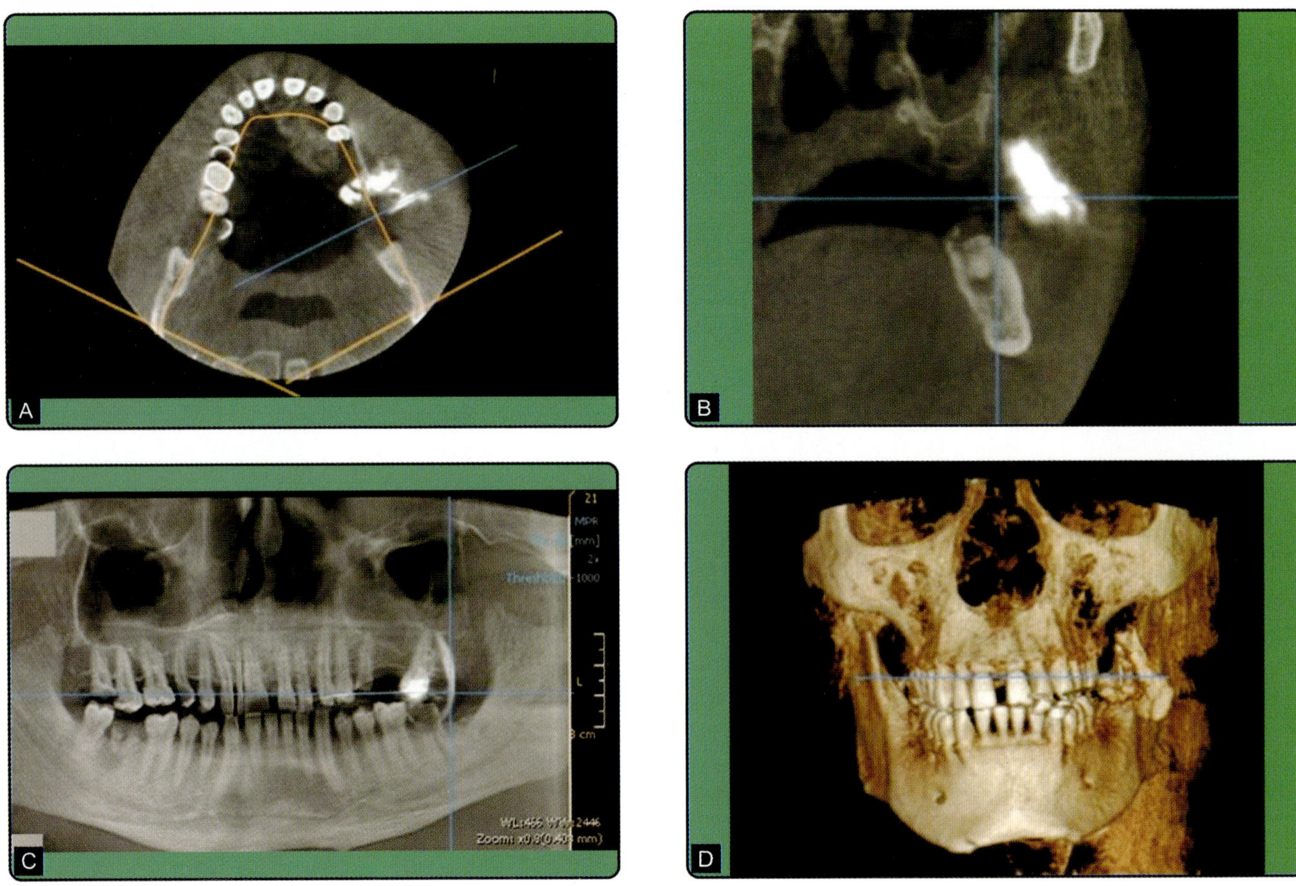

Figures 8.25A to D: Axial view. **A.** Coronal; **B.** Panoramic; **C.** Three-dimensional (3D) reconstruction; **D.** Images of cone beam computed tomography sialography in a case of lymphoepithelial lesion showing unspecific accumulation of contrast medium.

REFERENCES

1. Hassan B, Jacobs R. Cone Beam Computed Tomography-3D Imaging in Oral and Maxillofacial Surgery. Touch briefings. 2008;38-40.
2. Suomalainen A, Ventä I, Mattila M, et al. Reliability of CBCT and other radiographic methods in preoperative evaluation of lower third molars. Oral Surg Oral Med Oral Pathol Oral Radiol Endod. 2010;109(2):276-84.
3. Kamrun N, Tetsumura A, Nomura Y, et al. Visualization of the superior and inferior borders of the mandibular canal: a comparative study using digital panoramic radiographs and cross-sectional computed tomography images. Oral Surg Oral Med Oral Pathol Oral Radiol. 2013;115(4):550-7.
4. Rood JP, Shehab BA. The radiological prediction of inferior alveolar nerve injury during third molar surgery. Br J Oral Maxillofac Surg. 1990;28(1):20-5.
5. Oberoi S, Knueppel S. Three-dimensional assessment of impacted canines and root resorption using cone beam computed tomography. Oral Surg Oral Med Oral Pathol Oral Radiol. 2012;113(2):260-7.
6. Ericson S, Kurol PJ. Resorption of incisors after ectopic eruption of maxillary canines: a CT study. Angle Orthod. 2000;70(6):415-23.
7. Liu DG, Zhang WL, Zhang ZY, et al. Three-dimensional evaluations of supernumerary teeth using cone-beam computed tomography for 487 cases. Oral Surg Oral Med Oral Pathol Oral Radiol Endod. 2007;103(3):403-11.
8. Scarfe WC. Imaging of maxillofacial trauma: evolutions and emerging revolutions. Oral Surg Oral Med Oral Pathol Oral Radiol Endod. 2005;100(2 Suppl):S75-96.
9. Kaeppler G, Cornelius CP, Ehrenfeld M, et al. Diagnostic efficacy of cone-beam computed tomography for mandibular fractures. Oral Surg Oral Med Oral Pathol Oral Radiol. 2013;116(1):98-104.
10. Closmann JJ, Schmidt BL. The use of cone beam computed tomography as an aid in evaluating and treatment planning for mandibular cancer. J Oral Maxillofac Surg. 2007;65(4):766-71.
11. Tetradis S, Anstey P, Graff-Radford S. Cone beam computed tomography in the diagnosis of dental disease. J Calif Dent Assoc. 2010;38(1):27-32.
12. Hendrikx AW, Maal T, Dieleman F, et al. Cone-beam CT in the assessment of mandibular invasion by oral squamous cell carcinoma: results of the preliminary study. Int J Oral Maxillofac Surg. 2010;39(5):436-9.
13. Shahidi S, Vojdani M, Paknahad M. Correlation between articular eminence steepness measured with cone-beam computed tomography and clinical dysfunction index in patients with temporomandibular joint dysfunction. Oral Surg Oral Med Oral Pathol Oral Radiol. 2013;116(1):91-7.
14. Honey OB, Scarfe WC, Hilgers MJ, et al. Accuracy of cone-beam computed tomography imaging of the temporomandibular joint: comparisons with panoramic radiology and linear tomography. Am J Orthod Dentofacial Orthop. 2007;132(4):429-38.
15. Zhang ZL, Cheng JG, Li G, et al. Measurement accuracy of temporomandibular joint space in Promax 3-dimensional cone-beam computerized tomography images. Oral Surg Oral Med Oral Pathol Oral Radiol. 2012;114(1):112-7.
16. Albuquerque MA, Gaia BF, Cavalcanti MG. Comparison between multislice and cone-beam computerized tomography in the volumetric assessment of cleft palate. Oral Surg Oral Med Oral Pathol Oral Radiol Endod. 2011;112(2):249-57.
17. van Loon B, Maal TJ, Plooij JM, et al. 3D Stereophotogrametric assessment of pre- and postoperative volumetric changes in the cleft lip and palate nose. Int J Oral Maxillofac Surg. 2010;39(6):534-40.
18. Abdel-Wahed N, Amer ME, Abo-Taleb NS. Assessment of the role of cone beam computed sialography in diagnosing salivary gland lesions. Imaging Science in Dentistry. 2013;43(1):17-23.
19. Ngu RK, Brown JE, Whaites EJ, et al. Salivary duct strictures: nature and incidence in benign salivary obstruction. Dentomaxillofac Radiol. 2007;36(2):63-7.
20. Li B, Long X, Cheng Y, et al. Cone beam CT sialography of Stafne bone cavity. Dentomaxillofac Radiol. 2011;40(8):519-23.
21. Jadu F, Yaffe MJ, Lam EW. A comparative study of the effective radiation doses from cone beam computed tomography and plain radiography for sialography. Dentomaxillofac Radiol. 2010;39(5):257-63.

9

Chapter

Role of Cone Beam Computed Tomography in Periodontal Disease

Pratik Dedhia

INTRODUCTION

A phenomenal and unprecedented interest in cone beam computed tomography (CBCT) from all fields of dentistry is currently underway. The CBCT has revolutionized maxillofacial imaging, facilitating the transition of dental diagnosis from two-dimensional (2D) to three-dimensional (3D) images and expanding the role of imaging from diagnosis to image guidance of operative and surgical procedures. Not only that we are able now to provide more accurate diagnosis with this imaging modality but also we are ably based on the new radiographic data to guide and assess various surgical and clinical interventions.

Studies have shown that early detection of periodontal disease is important in the prevention of tooth loss and/or for the patient's general health. However, current diagnostic approaches including clinical probing and intraoral radiography have shown several limitations in their reliability. Clinical probing is dependent on the probing force, while periapical radiographs or bitewings may over- or under-estimate the amount of bone loss due to projection errors. One of the main drawbacks of intraoral radiography is the overlap of anatomical structures and lack of 3D information. This often hinders a true distinction between the buccal and lingual cortical plate, and complicates the evaluation of periodontal bone defects, especially the infrabony lesions, also denoted as craters and furcation involvements. The application of CBCT imaging with a combination of existing 2D digital intraoral radiographs may offer new perspectives on periodontal diagnosis and treatment planning.

Cone beam computed tomography can be used in assessing a detailed morphologic description of the bone, because it has proved to be accurate with only minimal error margins. The measurements proved to be as accurate as direct measurements with a periodontal probe. Furthermore, it also aids in assessing furcation involvements. CBCT can be used to detect buccal and lingual defects, which was previously not possible with conventional 2D radiographs. Additionally, owing to the high accuracy of CBCT measurements, intrabony defects can accurately be measured and dehiscence, fenestration defects and periodontal cysts assessed. CBCT has also proved its superiority in evaluating the outcome of regenerative periodontal therapy.

The reported applications of CBCT in periodontology are for diagnostic and treatment outcome evaluations of periodontitis.

CBCT IN ASSESSMENT OF PERIODONTAL LIGAMENT SPACE

The earliest signs of periodontal disease in radiographs are fuzziness; break in the continuity of lamina dura and a wedge-shaped radiolucent area at the mesial and distal aspect of the periodontal ligament (PDL) space. In addition to this, the proper observation of PDL space may offer some potential regarding detection of occlusal trauma and the effects of systemic diseases on the periodontium.

CBCT FOR PERIODONTAL DEFECT MEASUREMENTS

Furcation Craters, Buccal and Lingual Defects

The extent of periodontal marginal bone loss is not always easy to determine and certainly not the extent with which furcation areas are involved. The CBCT images provide better diagnostic and quantitative information on periodontal bone levels in three dimensions than conventional radiography. The CBCT is found to be as accurate as direct measurements using a periodontal probe and as reliable as radiographs for interproximal areas. Although, 2D radiography is of use for interproximal lesions, its limitation was anticipated during early investigations, determining its diagnostic value for periapical and periodontal disease. So, when buccal and lingual defects cannot be diagnosed with radiography, CBCT is a superior technique (Figs 9.1 to 9.3A to E).[1-5] Periodontal defects in human dry cadaver skulls using CBCT and traditional methods revealed that there was no difference between intraoral radiography and CBCT in linear measurements for all defects. In another study, researchers evaluated accuracy and reliability of CBCT for measuring alveolar bone height and detecting bony dehiscence and fenestration. The CBCT measurements were found to be equivalent to direct measurements and dehiscences were diagnosed with higher accuracy than fenestrations. The CBCT and multislice computed tomography (MSCT) images were used for alveolar bone width measurements. There was no significant difference between the measurements obtained by CBCT and MSCT or direct measurements and radiographic methods.

Furcation involvement is one of the major problems in the treatment of periodontal disease and is directly associated with tooth loss. Therefore, furcation lesions must be detected with accuracy at an early stage of the disease. Periapical and interproximal intraoral radiographs are widely accepted as valuable tools for establishing the diagnosis and guiding the treatment of periodontal disease, mainly to assess the pattern and extent of bone resorption. These characteristics can be clearly viewed in the interproximal alveolar bone. However, intraoral radiographs have the inherent inaccuracy of a 2D examination. This is clearly overcome by CBCT imaging.

Cone beam computed tomography images of maxillary molars provide detailed information of furcation involvement and a reliable basis for treatment decision. Intrasurgical furcation involvement measurements were compared by using CBCT images and periapical radiography, and it was reported that CBCT images demonstrated a high accuracy in assessing the loss of periodontal tissue and classifying the degree of furcation involvement in maxillary molars.

The CBCT provides substantial additional information about the root morphology and the residual attachment of maxillary molars. These CBCT-derived data can help in understanding the severity and morphology of bony defects of the furcation lesion, and provide more evidence for periodontal diagnosis and treatment planning.

A study on the use of CBCT to examine the geometric relationship between the roots and furcation areas of the mandibular first molars has verified that the X-ray beam projection angle affects the accuracy and diagnosis of a furcation defect (Figs 9.4A and B). Changes in horizontal angulations cause geometric distortion in intraoral radiography.[6]

SOFT TISSUE CBCT FOR THE MEASUREMENT OF GINGIVAL TISSUE AND THE DIMENSIONS OF THE DENTOGINGIVAL UNIT

The novel method is based on CBCT technology, called soft tissue CBCT (ST-CBCT), to visualize and precisely measure distances corresponding to the hard and soft tissues of the periodontium and dentogingival attachment apparatus. With this simple and non-invasive technique, clinicians are able to determine the relationships between:

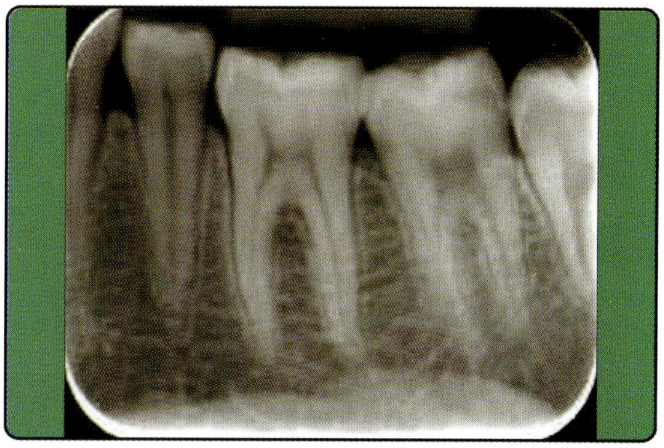

Figure 9.1: Intraoral periapical radiograph of mandibular molar region

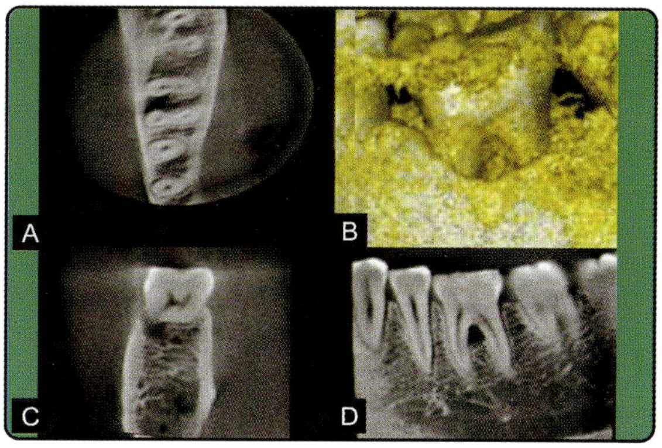

Figures 9.2A to D: Cone beam computed tomography (CBCT) images of mandibular first molar showing the marginal bone defect and the precisely assessed degree of bone loss; in the upper right corner is a 3D image based on the radiographic volume data. **A.** Axial view showing bone loss in furcation region; **B.** 3D reconstruction demonstrating bone loss in furcation region; **C.** Cross-sectional image showing bone loss around first molar; **D.** Periapical radiograph showing bone loss in furcation region with lack of details on quantity and type of bone loss.

1. Gingival margin and the facial bone crest.
2. Gingival margin and the cementoenamel junction (CEJ).
3. The CEJ and facial bone crest.

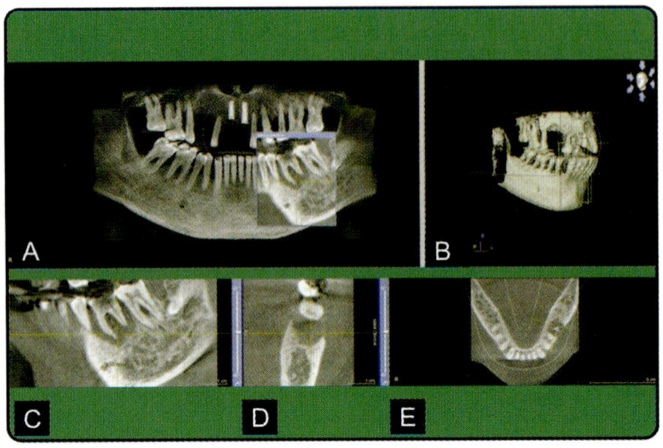

Figures 9.3A to E: Extend of the endo-perio lesion associated with left mandibular right molar demonstrated accurately on cone beam computed tomography (CBCT) images. **A.** Orthopantomogram (OPG) showing endo-perio lesion in left first mandibular molar; **B.** 3D reconstruction; **C.** Sagittal view showing extend of bone loss; **D.** Cross-sectional image showing bone loss around first molar on buccal and lingual side; **E.** Axial view showing endo-perio lesion with loss of buccal cortical plates.

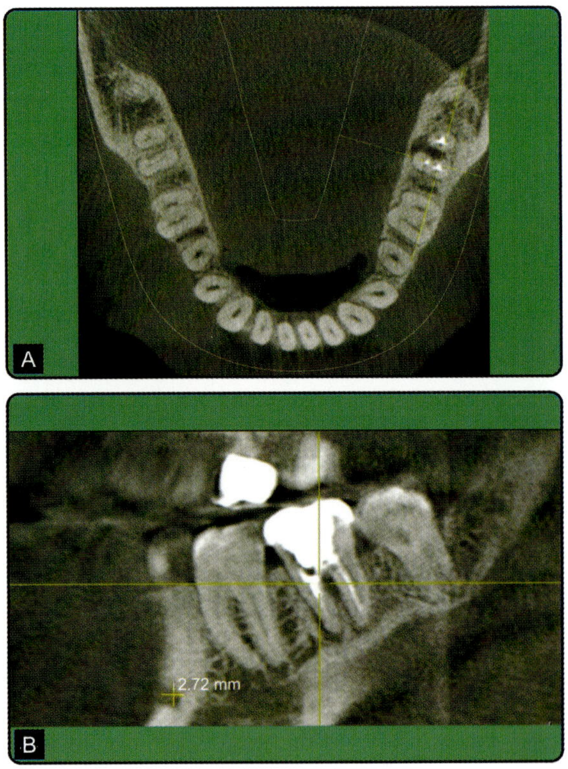

Figures 9.4A and B: Furcation involvement with mandibular left second molar seen on axial and sagittal cone beam computed tomography (CBCT) images. **A.** Axial view showing bone loss in furcation region of mandibular left second molar; **B.** Sagittal view showing bone loss in furcation region.

The width of the facial and palatal/lingual alveolar bone and the width of the facial and palatal/lingual gingival also could be measured (Figs 9.5A to C and 9.6).[7]

Tissue biotypes have been linked to the outcomes of periodontal and implant therapy. When tissue biotypes of 22 fresh cadaver heads were assessed clinically and radiographically with CBCT scans, the labial gingival thickness was moderately associated with the underlying bone thickness measured with CBCT. These measurements were an accurate representation of the clinical thickness of both labial gingiva and alveolar bone.[8] The ST-CBCT will certainly aid clinicians in the planning and execution of a number of procedures in dentistry with increased predictability.

CBCT PRECISION IN ALVEOLAR BONE DENSITY MEASUREMENT

Radiographic follow-up of bone healing after grafting is challenging because of the overlapping of gaining and losing areas within the graft. The new volumetric imaging method, CBCT, offers an opportunity to see inside the bone, and pinpoint and measure densities in small localized areas such as a vertical periodontal defect or an alveolar bone graft. This precision would make it possible to reproducibly quantify the bone remodeling after bone grafting.

CBCT IN GUIDED TISSUE REGENERATION THERAPY

Evidence suggests that guided tissue regeneration (GTR) therapy with a barrier membrane can successfully treat intrabony defects.[9-12] The purpose of placing materials over intrabony defects is to keep the gingival epithelium and connective tissue away from the root surface, while bone is being regenerated. Currently, non-absorbable expanded polytetrafluoroethylene (ePTFE) and absorbable membranes are used as barriers in GTR therapy. These barriers are preformed into various sizes and shapes to fit periodontal defects of different morphologies and in different locations. For GTR therapy to be successful, tight fitting of the membrane to the root surface and complete coverage of the bone defect are important.[13] However, most membranes must be individually trimmed and adjusted to fit the root, and cover the bone defect. In particular, when a GTR membrane is placed in an interproximal area, the bone defects complicate the adjustment of the GTR membrane, thus prolonging the operation. The CBCT visualizes the morphology of bone defects and furcation involvement, and the data are easily converted into 3D images.[14-19]

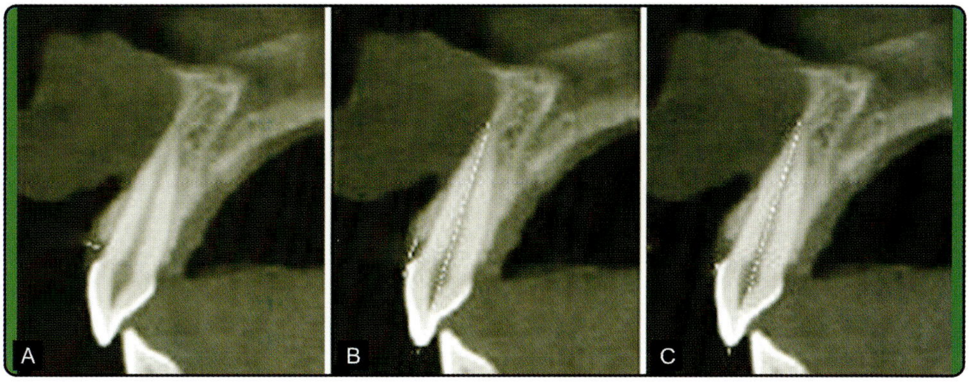

Figures 9.5A to C: Soft tissue cone beam computed tomography scan. **A.** Measurement of the thickness of the facial gingiva performed on the image of the patient with a thick periodontal biotype; **B.** Measurement of the distance of the gingival margin to the facial bone crest; **C.** Measurement of the distance of the gingival margin to the cementoenamel junction (dotted lines represent the long axis of the tooth).

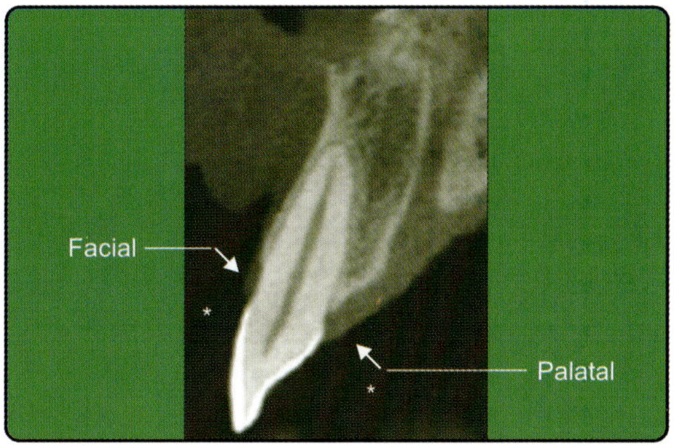

Figure 9.6: Image of the soft tissue cone beam computed tomography scan showing a dark space (asterisks) on the facial and palatal/lingual aspects, allowing the clear visualization of the facial (arrow) and palatal (arrowhead) gingiva.

In a study done by Masatoshi T et al,[20] they have used CBCT for diagnosis of angular bone defects. They used only the axial image to make a template for the GTR membrane using transparency film, which can be sterilized before surgery. This basic and clinical study confirmed that, by using the template, the membrane can be easily trimmed and adapted to the root surface in either the maxillary or mandibular arch. In contrast, without the use of CT, their basic study showed that the membrane had a larger interproximal area and was smaller at the mesial buccal site. Furthermore, the membrane trimming time was shown to be shortened using computed tomography (CT). Also, a 4–6 mm clinical attachment gain and an improved condition of the hard tissues, after 6–18 months was observed, which may have been the result of optimal membrane adaptation and accurate diagnosis of bone defects using CBCT. Furthermore, no membrane exposure was encountered. Membrane exposure results in bacterial contamination, which may impair successful regeneration. Ability to select the optimal shape and size of the membrane might decrease the chance of membrane exposure during the healing period. Thus, this procedure may prove to be a useful aid to periodontal examination and diagnosis, and for predicting and evaluating the outcome of periodontal regenerative treatment.

As CBCT scanning is finding more and more applications in dentomaxillofacial radiology, it stands as the privileged field of imaging in periodontics. Current methods of detecting alveolar bone level changes over time or determining 3D architecture of osseous defects are inadequate. This issue has been addressed by the recent low-cost CBCT machines, which has resulted in production of an affordable, low-radiation high-quality 3D data. The CBCT is an essential diagnostic tool also for selection of implant design and its placement. It provides high quality of diagnostic images that have an absorbed dose that is comparable with other dental surveys and less than a conventional CT, and thus following the principles of radiation protection to reduce the radiations 'as low as reasonably achievable' (ALARA).

CONCLUSION

The CBCT with its high spatial resolution, affordability, smaller size, lower acquisition and maintenance have made it as a natural fit in periodontal imaging.

REFERENCES

1. Mengel R, Candir M, Shiratori K, et al. Digital volume tomography in the diagnosis of periodontal defects: an in vitro study on native pig and human mandibles. J Periodontol. 2005;76(5):665-73.

2. Misch KA, Yi ES, Sarment DP. Accuracy of cone beam computed tomography for periodontal defect measurements. J Periodontol. 2006;77(7):1261-6.
3. Vandenberghe B, Jacobs R, Yang J. Diagnostic validity (or acuity) of 2D CCD versus 3D CBCT-images for assessing periodontal breakdown. Oral Surg Oral Med Oral Pathol Oral Radiol Endod. 2007;104(3):395-401.
4. Mol A, Balasundaram A. In vitro cone beam computed tomography imaging of periodontal bone. Dentomaxillofac Radiol. 2008;37(6):319-24.
5. Vandenberghe B, Jacobs R, Yang J. Detection of periodontal bone loss using digital intraoral and cone beam computed tomography images: an in vitro assessment of bony and/or infrabony defects. Dentomaxillofac Radiol. 2008;37(5):252-60.
6. Hishikawa T, Izumi M, Naitoh M, et al. The effect of horizontal X-ray beam angulation on the detection of furcation defects of mandibular first molars in intraoral radiography. Dentomaxillofac Radiol. 2010;39(2):85-90.
7. Januario AL, Barriviera M, Duarte WR. Soft tissue cone-beam computed tomography: a novel method for the measurement of gingival tissue and the dimensions of the dentogingival unit. J Esthet Restor Dent. 2008;20(6):366-73.
8. Fu JH, Yeh CY, Chan HL, et al. Tissue biotype and its relation to the underlying bone morphology. J Periodontol. 2010;81(4):569-74.
9. Cortellini P, Pini Prato G, Tonetti MS. Periodontal regeneration of human infrabony defects. I. Clinical measures. J Periodontol. 1993;64(4):254-60.
10. McClain PK, Schallhorn RG. Long-term assessment of combined osseous composite grafting, root conditioning, and guided tissue regeneration. Int J Periodontics Restorative Dent. 1993;13(1):9-27.
11. Becker W, Becker BE, Berg L, et al. New attachment after treatment with root isolation procedure: report for treated Class III and Class II furcations and vertical osseous defects. Int J Periodontics Restorative Dent. 1998;8(3):8-23.
12. Handelsman M, Davarpanah M, Celletti R. Guided tissue regeneration with and without citric acid treatment in vertical osseous defects. Int J Periodontics Restorative Dent. 1991;11(5):350-63.
13. Becker W, Becker BE. Clinical application of guided tissue regeneration: surgical considerations. Periodontol 2000. 1993;1:46-53.
14. Ramachandran GN, Lakshminarayanan AV. Three-dimensional reconstruction from radiographs and electron micrographs: application convolutions instead of Fourier tranforms. Proc Natl Acad Sci U S A. 1971;68(9):2236-40.
15. Hounsfield GN. Computerized transverse axial scanning (tomography). 1. Description of system. Br J Radiol. 1973;46(552):1016-22.
16. Marsh JL, Vannier MW. The 'third' dimension in craniofacial surgery. Plast Reconstr Surg. 1983;71(6):759-67.
17. Mutoh Y, Ohashi Y, Uchiyama N, et al. Three-dimensional analysis of condylar hyperplasia with computed tomography. J Craniomaxillofac Surg. 1991;19(2):49-55.
18. Vannier MW, Hildebolt CF, Conover G, et al. Three-dimensional dental imaging by spiral CT. A progress report. Oral Surg Oral Med Oral Pathol Oral Radiol Endod. 1997;84(5):561-70.
19. Ito K, Yoshinuma N, Goke E, et al. Clinical application of a new compact computed tomography system for evaluating the outcome of regenerative therapy: a case report. J Periodontol. 2001;72(5):696-702.
20. Takane M, Sato S, Suzuki K, et al. Clinical application of cone beam computed tomography for ideal absorbable membrane placement in interproximal bone defects. J Oral Sci. 2010;52(1):63-9.

10 Chapter

Future of Cone Beam Computed Tomography

Yoshinori Arai, Prashant P Jaju

INTRODUCTION

Teleradiology field is growing tremendously due to limited numbers of oral maxillofacial radiologists trained in interpreting in CBCT images. Now CBCT data can be transferred via cloud, stored and interpreted by oral radiologists at distant location and reports are made available to dentists and patients within few hours. This chapter highlights the future role of CBCT in teleradiology and its future applications.

DIGITAL IMAGING AND COMMUNICATION IN MEDICINE

The digital imaging and communication in medicine (DICOM) is a standard for handling, storing, printing and transmitting information in medical imaging. A DICOM file contains a patient's X-ray image or series of images and other patient-related information (e.g. patient name, identification number and acquisition modality) as selected from a library of standardized terms. The DICOM library is extensive and continually updated to reflect changing identification standards. The DICOM files are fully encrypted to allow safe electronic communication over the internet. With this conversion from legacy to digital imaging have emerged the need for a software strategy that allows the communication of patient, diagnostic and other acquisition data along with the imaging information. The DICOM standards were first developed by the American College of Radiology and National Electrical Manufacturers Association. These standards are regularly revised to improve compatibility with electronic records and improve clinical workflow in the medical environment. By using a standardized format, the images and associated data can be viewed regardless of the proprietary acquisition modality that was used to take the imaging study, allowing for cross-vendor interoperability or connectivity. Dentists are also able to communicate with their medical colleagues via Health Insurance Portability and Accountability Act (HIPAA) compliant internet connections. Dentistry has been actively involved in formulation of DICOM standards since 1996, when the American Dental Association joined the DICOM committee. As a result, DICOM standards began to include definitions for image objects with special categorization for intraoral projections and color photography. Today, most companies producing imaging devices (termed acquisition modalities) include DICOM image identification.

Digital imaging is increasingly used for evaluation of dental caries, oral pathology presurgical and preorthodontic treatment assessment.[1]

Numerous software systems [termed picture archiving and communications system (PACS)] have been developed to allow for the storage, retrieval and viewing of digital DICOM images. Much work still needs to be done before dentistry is fully integrated with respect to DICOM. For example, DICOM images need to be integrated with many electronic dental record software products currently available. In February 2010, the DICOM group that represents the dentistry specialty met to discuss issues related to the DICOM standards including the use of imaging in diagnosis, treatment simulation, treatment guidance and tissue restoration.[2]

In DICOM terminology, the device used to take an image is called acquisition modality. Interoperability is important for an acquisition modality; it should be fully functional and operate without glitches. Theoretically, all devices should be able to connect with any other DICOM-compliant product; this is outlined in the conformance statement.

The DICOM conformance statement should contain the information necessary for technical use, when modalities are connected. The DICOM performance statements for various acquisition modalities and other connected machines are typically available for download on the manufacturer's website. The conformance statements for acquisition devices are standardized to allow comparison of DICOM devices from different manufacturers. The DICOM conformance statement is simply a diagram that demonstrates. For example, a digital dental X-ray taken by a specific intraoral imaging product will be downloaded to another vendor's server and then displayed properly on another company's computer monitor.

Acquisition Devices

An acquisition device is any instrument that produces a digitized image including computed tomography (CT), magnetic resonance imaging (MRI), ultrasound, digital projection radiography and X-ray machines that allow periapical, panoramic or cephalometric imaging. Dental digital imaging also includes three-dimensional (3D) CT, digital photography and digitally driven computer-aided design/computer-aided manufacturing (CAD/CAM) systems. Generally, newer standard dental digital imaging equipment [e.g. intraoral digital X-ray systems, panoramic imaging, cone beam CT (CBCT)] is DICOM compliant. However, the standards for DICOM compliance for some devices, including 3D computed tomography and CAD/CAM systems, as well as interoperability with respect to PACS, have not yet been established.

Most medical centers and large physician-based health management organizations use PACS to manage digital DICOM files including acquisition, storage, retrieval and viewing. In dentistry, the use of PACS is primarily limited to academic centers and dental clinics in large hospital facilities, where there is need for transmission of data between departments. In these settings, the use of DICOM-compliant imaging is critical for a number of reasons including HIPAA compliance. A review article by Grauer et al described DICOM as it relates to CBCT images in orthodontics, the measurement of CBCT images, the creation of two-dimensional (2D) radiographs from DICOM CBCT files, segmentation engines and multimodal images, the registration and superimposition of 3D images, special applications for quantitative analysis and 3D surgical prediction. Most sophisticated software applications allow the transformation of images along different planes. They also allow visualization of a specific region of interest at different angles and the scaling of sections, as desired. Although, rendering images for qualitative assessment is appropriate in 2D imaging, quantitative assessment in 3D rendering has limitations. For example, most landmarks visualized in 2D either cannot be visualized or are difficult to locate on a curved 3D surface. In addition, a rendered image is impacted by many factors including contrast, movement during acquisition, the presence of metal, signal-to-noise ratio and the threshold filters that have been applied by the operator. Thus, it is recommended that landmarks need to be located within a stack of slices. With respect to accuracy and reliability of measurements on CBCT images, there may be differences depending on the way landmarks are located within the slices.[3]

A DICOM 3D software system has not yet been linked to diagnosis classification. In addition, some of the available tools have not yet been validated with respect to accuracy and precision. Therefore, the data included on a DICOM file should be interpreted with caution. Implant planning may also use DICOM-compliant imaging. In one study, data from a CT taken with an intraoral template in place was stored on a compact disk read-only memory (CD-ROM) in DICOM format and then uploaded into an implant software program, where it was then used to calculate parameters necessary for site preparation. The authors noted that this approach may improve surgical accuracy, particularly for regions where exactness is important such as in cases where anatomical sites have little space (e.g. atrophic maxillae) or where there have been sinus lifts necessitating a zygomatic approach. To establish accuracy during the actual procedure, infrared light-emitting diodes were connected to rotatory instruments and to the patient's template, then viewed in real time on a monitor. Such computer-assisted navigation systems are in development, but DICOM connectivity issues have yet to be resolved.[3]

Two other areas of dental application related to DICOM are oral surgery and the diagnosis of dental caries. With respect to oral surgery, DICOM files offer considerable information that is useful in diagnosis and surgical planning. However, some evidence suggests that the complexity of the DICOM file data may be problematic in research. A study exploring CBCT-based DICOM files and the properties of these images used to evaluate maxillofacial bone grafts suggested that DICOM files can be used in research looking at issues associated with graft viability, but that the parameters associated with these files may hinder comparison of results between studies, thus compromising their scientific impact. Two innovations in DICOM and PACS implementation include use of the internet for image transfer and a mobile device as a viewer. The PACS systems allowing DICOM images to be sent via the internet represent a significant step forward in the communication of digital files. Using the internet, a clinician with proper identification can access the clinic's PACS server upload and display a patient imaging file (using the unique identifier attributed to the DICOM file), while at a distant satellite clinic or other remote location. Recent advances in the digital display capabilities of mobile devices, including tablets, dramatically increases the clinical possibilities associated with internet-based image transfer. Internet-based electronic dental records delivery is also currently available, but these software systems may not in all cases, be fully integrated with DICOM imaging solutions.

Future work is to include the development of guidelines for standardization of digital photographic structured displays for both intraoral and extraoral projections, the creation of templates for reports, the development of guidelines for presentation states including overlays used in dentistry and surgical workflow issues within DICOM used in dental implantology.

Picture Archiving and Communication Systems/Radiographic Information System and Radiographic Information Delivery

The PACS have been developed and used in medicine for many years for the ability to store, retrieve and share image information between medical ground and entire industry. Until now, dentistry had only a couple of such products and they were not widely used. Indeed, in the best of world's medical and dental records could be shared and distributed using PACS systems.

Radiographic IC formation system (RIS) IS is really just the information highway to deliver the radiologist's report to the referring hospital, clinician or colleague. The two systems or products really go hand in hand. Now there is a PACS/RIS product specifically for dentistry. CyberMed's OnDemand PACS/RIS was designed to handle the necessary data volumes, deliver reports and analyses, and archive client data off-site, which was one of the many necessary HIPAA regulations. Till date, it is the only HIPAA-compliant product used for CBCT volumes. Each patient file ranges from 60 to 300 MB. These large files must be moved quickly, safely and efficiently without corruption. Dentistry has truly 'made it to the big time' with this capability.

Image to Device Processes

Perhaps the most exciting area of dental and maxillofacial imaging will be fabrication of radiographic stents, surgical guides, study and orthodontic models and other devices directly from their office computers. Companies are currently

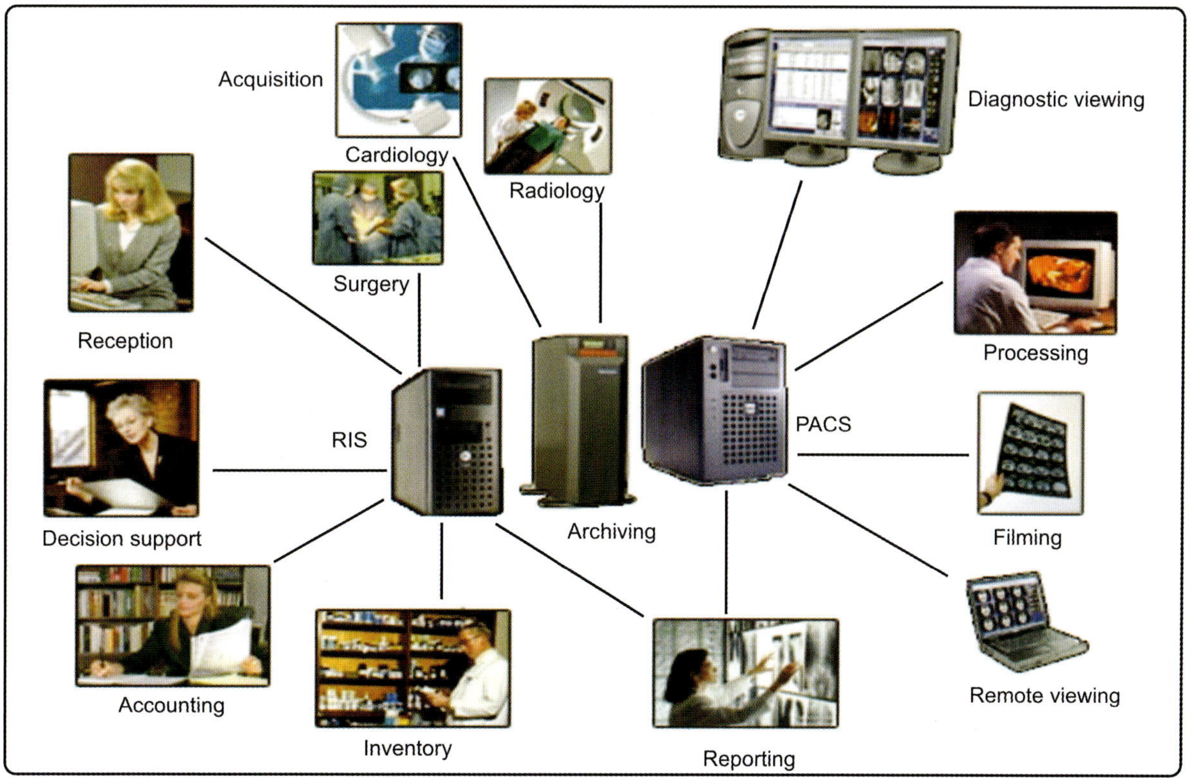

Figure 10.1: Workflow of picture archiving and communication systems (PACS)/radiographic information system (RIS)and radiographic information delivery

raising venture capital to deliver these appliances and devices electronically. The cone beam image data makes this possible. Already we can see the patient's 3D color dentition. Many clinicians are sending their patient's data for surgical guide construction through companies like Nobel Biocare. Larger surgical guides, requiring temporary horizontal 'anchorage' to place multiple fixtures for overdentures can be received by mail or courier delivery. But, many more services, including faster and simpler delivery for single implant cases, will soon be offered through 'internet portals' or distributive networks because of CBCT imaging (Fig. 10.1).[4]

SOFTWARE IMPROVEMENTS

Software from the machine manufacturers is always good. They could not have introduced their hardware without accompanying software and be successful. However, some of the manufacturers have proprietary software. Examples are Imaging Sciences International (i-CAT, Hatfield, Pennsylvania) and AFP Imaging (NewTom 3G and VG, Elmsford, New York). Although, both these machines, as all other CBCT machines, scan and export their volume data to third party software, DICOM data cannot be imported into the manufacturer's software for use with their templates and reporting tools. Although, not a serious drawback, it is a point to consider, when purchasing or using these machines. The most robust type of 3D color software would include several parameters to assign to the voxel information. Every manufacturer and third-party software can handle the 2D grayscale assignment to the voxel. Some even have algorithms to approximate Hounsfield units (HU). Some third-party software can also perform surface rendering of the voxel units assigning a color to the voxel.

A few vendors, for example, Planmeca (Romexis, Helsinki, Finland) and Imaging Sciences International (3DVR, Hatfield, Pennsylvania), and can assign a transparency value to each voxel to make a seemingly 'transparent' image. A third-party company, Anatomage (San Jose, California) has this type of software and has created products for cephalometric landmark AnatoCeph tracing and implant planning (InVivoDental software, Anatomage Inc, San Jose, California). The highest level of software treatment is able to assign color, transparency and opacity values to the cone beam volumetric tomography (CBVT) voxel information. To date, only OnDemand 3D (CyberMed International, Seoul, Korea) can perform these tasks (Table 10.1).[4]

Table 10.1: Third-party softwares[4]

Manufacturer	Product name	Primary software tasks
3dMD	3dMD face 3dMD cranial	Orthodontics
Anatomage	InVivoDental AnatoCeph	Implant Orthodontics
CyberMed	OnDemand 3D Vworks	Multiple
Dolphin	Dolphin 3D	Orthodontics
Nobel Biocare	NobelGuide	Implant
Materialise dental	SimPlant	Implant
3Diemme	3Diagnosys	Multiple

Useful Software Improvements

- All software will be able to assign all three attributes namely color, transparency and opacity (Figs 10.2A and B)
- Improved 'scatter rejection' algorithms
- All software completely DICOM compliant
- Software in four dimensions to create the 'virtual articulator'

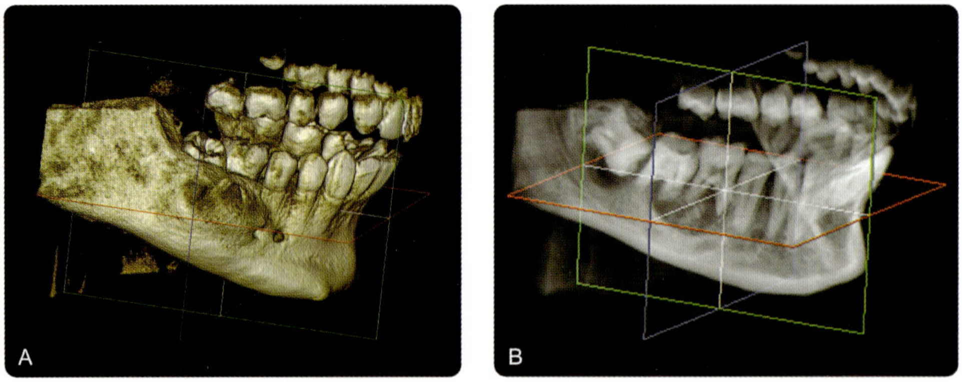

Figures 10.2A and B: Third-party software rendering three-dimensional reconstruction in transparency, opacity and color. **A.** Three-dimensional reconstruction via third party software having bone window; **B.** Three-dimensional reconstruction via third party software having X-ray window.

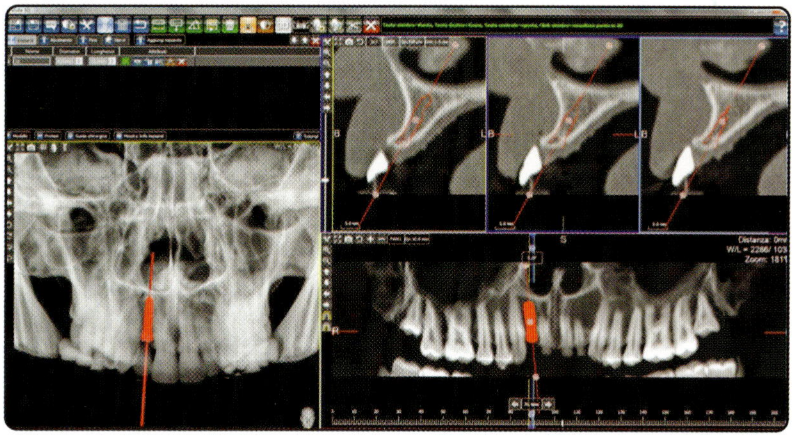

Figure 10.3: Virtual implant planning with third-party software (3Diagnosys; 3Diemme, Italy)

- Online, internet 'portal' software to speed surgical guide construction and delivery as well as interpretive reports, and analytic images (e.g. measured implant sites) (Figs 10.3 and 10.4)
- The PACS/RIS systems for dentistry.

FUTURE OF CONE BEAM COMPUTED TOMOGRAPHY MACHINES

There have always been two traditional methods for dental radiology; panoramic radiography and intraoral radiography. Panoramic radiography utilizes curved tomography and is exclusively used for dentistry. Intraoral radiography was very unique. The film is inserted into the oral cavity and it achieves the highest resolution. These two unique methods are in daily use in dentistry. Since 2001, two types of CBCT have entered dental imaging market. One type CBCT is like panoramic radiography and cephalography, whose images cover large area. Therefore the radiation dose is higher than conventional radiography. In the future, medical CT will be upgraded and improvised for dental use along with a low radiation dose. This might lead to replacement of large volume CBCT by medical CT.

The other type of CBCT is the intraoral radiography that is limited area and high resolution CBCT. This system cannot be replaced by medical CT. This type of CBCT will be popular like traditional panoramic radiography (Fig. 10.5). We think that there will be limited volume CBCT at 50% dental clinic in the future.

Thinking of 'Image Gently' is very important (www.imagegently.org). We have to diagnose correctly and at the same time, we have to make the radiation dose as low as possible. If a limited area is chosen, the radiation dose can be reduced. However, there is one problem, the positioning is difficult for small areas. If the positioning is incorrect we have to expose the patient for a second time. This is stressful for the patient and the dentist. Therefore, the positioning system is important. In the future, the CBCT will be required to be user-friendly.

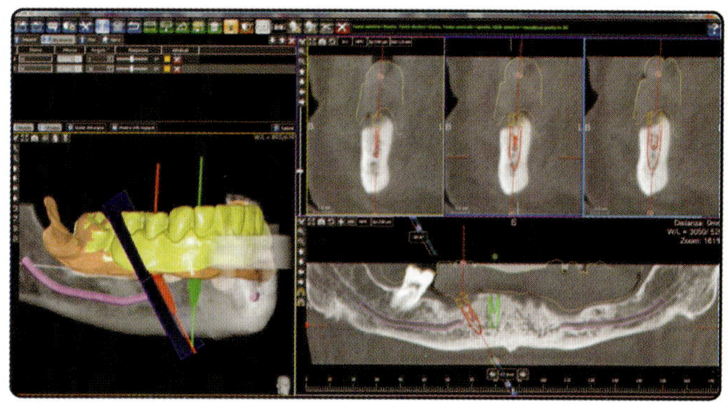

Figure 10.4: Virtual implant planning with third-party software assisting in computer-guided surgery (3Diagnosys; 3Diemme, Italy)

The life expectancy and reliability of the equipment are very important. Panoramic radiography units have used for over 15 years. So, CBCT units will need to perform reliably for a similar time. The CBCT will be able to develop for long lifetime (Box 10.1).

If we need 3D images for dental arch, we choose about 10 cm diameter FOV as cylinder. But there are problems with increase in radiation dose. To solve this, and fix the problem, a type of dental arch FOV was developed (Fig. 10.6). In this system, the X-ray is exposed along only the dental arch. Then the radiation dose can be reduced at soft tissue outside the dental arch region. In the future, other new dose reduction methods will be developed and become common place.

It can reduce the radiation dose at soft tissue outside of around dental arch region. Then that is reduced about 20% than conventional CBCT.

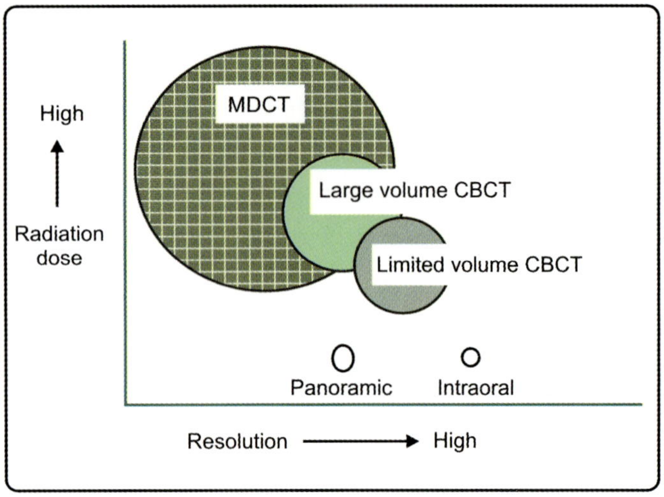

Figure 10.5: Resolution and radiation dose for each equipment (CBCT, cone beam computed tomography; MDCT, multidetector computed tomography).

Box 10.1: Future requirement of cone beam computed tomography machines
Limited area and high resolution
Low radiation
Easy positioning
Long lifetime
High reliability
Dental arch field of view

We wish to invent equipment, which delivers lower radiation dose, higher resolution, which is more user -friendly and has longer lifetime and higher reliability.

Future Studies on CBCT

With CBCT entering into the diagnostic and treatment modality of dental field, there is a continuous ongoing research into various unexplored applications, which will further enhance the utility of CBCT in dentistry. Current research projects on CBCT include the following:

1. Reliability of 3D cephalometric tracings on CBCT with 2D cephalometric tracings.[5]
2. Conversion of gray values obtained from CBCT machines into HU with various mathematical algorithms. This will ensure that CBCT will provide adequate HU values important for implant planning.[6]
3. Cervical vertebrae geometry assessment on CBCT to detect skeletal maturity.[7]
4. Methods to reduce metal artifacts from CBCT images.[8]

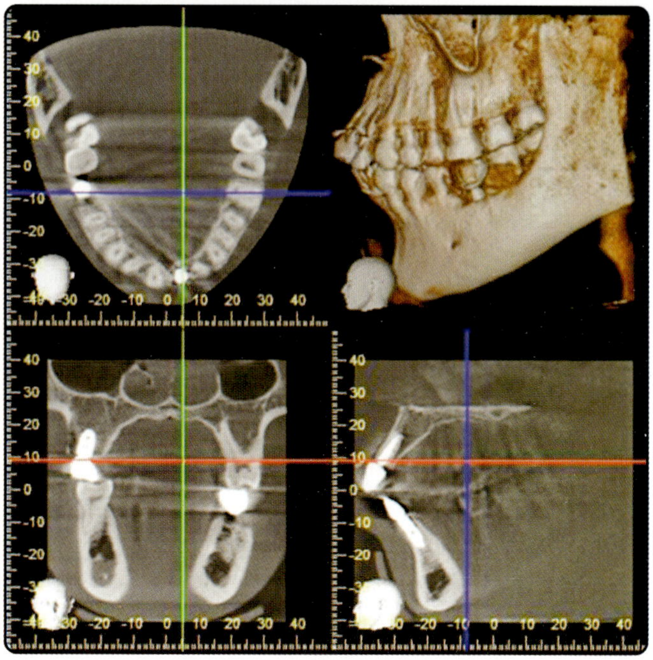

Figure 10.6: Dental arch field of view (FOV) (Veraviewepocs 3D R100, J morita, Kyoto, Japan)

5. The CBCT in dental caries diagnosis compared with intraoral radiographs.[9]
6. Methods to reduce the radiation dose during CBCT scans.[10]

CONCLUSION

Teleradiology, software and hardware improvements in CBCT technology will be the next step toward digital dentistry. But this is only possible with rational and selective application of CBCT thereby following the principle of image gently and reducing unnecessary radiation exposure to patients.

REFERENCES

1. Hellèn-Halme K, Nilsson M, Petersson A. Effect of monitors on approximal caries detection in digital radiographs—standard versus precalibrated DICOM part 14 displays: an in vitro study. Oral Surg Oral Med Oral Pathol Oral Radiol Endod. 2009;107(5):716-20.
2. Farman AG. The future of X-ray imaging in dentistry. Health Imaging Hub. [online]. Available from http://dental.healthimaginghub.com/portals/dental-pacs-news-article/2219-dicom-the-future-of-x-ray-imaging-in-dentistry. html [Accessed January 14, 2012].
3. Grauer D, Cevidanes LS, Proffit WR. Working with DICOM craniofacial images. Am J Orthod Dentofacial Orthop. 2009;136(3):460-70.

4. Miles DA. The future of dental and maxillofacial imaging. Dent Clin North Am. 2008;52(4):917-28.
5. Bholsithi W, Tharanon W, Chintakanon, et al. 3D vs. 2D cephalometric analysis comparisons with repeated measurements from 20 Thai males and 20 Thai females. Biomed Imaging Interv J. 2009;5(4):e21.
6. Molteni R. Prospects and challenges of rendering tissue density in Hounsfield units for cone beam computed tomography. Oral Surg Oral Med Oral Pathol Oral Radiol. 2013;116(1):105-19.
7. Santiago RC, Cunha AR, Junior GC, et al. New software for cervical vertebral geometry assessment and its relationship to skeletal maturation—a pilot study. Dentomaxillofac Radiol. 2014;43(2):20130238.
8. Bechara BB, Moore WS, McMahan CA, et al. Metal artefact reduction with cone beam CT: an in vitro study. Dentomaxillofac Radiol. 2012;41(3):248-53.
9. Park YS, Ahn JS, Kwon HB, et al. Current status of dental caries diagnosis using cone beam computed tomography. Imaging Sci Dent. 2011;41(2):43-51.
10. Güldner C, Ningo A, Voigt J, et al. Potential of dosage reduction in cone-beam computed tomography (CBCT) for radiological diagnostics of the paranasal sinuses. Eur Arch Otorhinolaryngol. 2013;270(4):1307-15.

11 Chapter

Role of Cone Beam Computed Tomography in Forensic Odontology

Sushma P Jaju

INTRODUCTION

Forensic dentistry or forensic odontology is the proper handling, examination and evaluation of dental evidence, which could be potentially utilized in human identification and in the interest of justice. The evidence that may be derived from teeth is the age (in children) and identification of the person to whom the teeth belong. This is done using dental records including radiographs, antemortem (prior to death) and postmortem photographs, and deoxyribonucleic acid (DNA). Forensic odontology is derived from Latin, meaning forum or where legal matters are discussed. Dental imaging plays a pivotal role in human identification in cases of natural calamities and criminal cases. Intraoral radiographs and panoramic radiographs have been routinely employed in forensic dentistry. With the advent of cone beam computed tomography (CBCT), forensic evaluation has received tremendous boost for human identification. Although the role of CBCT in forensic dentistry is still in nascent stage, but results hold promise and a definite role in near future.

CBCT IN DENTAL AGE ESTIMATION

Dental age estimation is important in both forensic and clinical work. In the forensic sciences, age information concerns living or deceased individuals and its estimation applies to criminal responsibility or marriage law. Birth data may also be lacking or dubious in questions of immigration and dental age can help in the determination of physiological age.[1] In clinical situations, dental age is of great interest to the pedodontist and orthodontist as it aids in diagnosis and the planning of treatment.[2]

Moreover, developing teeth are used as maturation indicators since they are less affected than other body tissues by endocrine diseases and environmental damage.[3]

Radiography is commonly used in estimating dental age. Two periods can be distinguished for dental age estimation—the first when the teeth are developing in the jaws and the second when all the teeth are fully formed. Intraoral and panoramic radiographs and the most common method for dental age assessment was first published by Demirjian et al.[1,2] In the second period, regressive age-related changes occurring in the fully grown teeth can be used as the basis of a scientific method.[1]

Radiographic methods based on correlations between age and ratios of the height and width of teeth, and the pulp cavity at various locations as measured on radiographs is the method of choice in regressive age-related changes in fully grown teeth. Panoramic radiographs and direct digital radiography systems have been widely used in nondestructive methods measuring the size of the dental pulp chamber and the proportion of secondary dentin deposit. However, these radiographic images are made from accumulated two-dimensional (2D) images of horizontal or parallel aspects of the tooth and, therefore, the ratios calculated by linear measurements never represent the entire three-dimensional (3D) morphological changes in teeth.[1]

At the present time, 3D digital tooth images can be acquired from living individuals using CBCT. Volumetric study by CBCT would be the best method according to Cameriere et al[4] but currently, it is generally not possible to apply it for dental age estimation only. However, as mentioned by Yang et al, the clinical introduction of CBCT has created new opportunities for obtaining 3D tooth radiographs, resulting in reasonable image quality at a low radiation dose.[5] Compared to microcomputed tomography, CBCT in dental use provides plenty of 3D volume information on the teeth in living individuals through a single scan of the target area.[1] Yang et al describe a first approach to age estimation by means of CBCT. Yang et al reported that, using their 3D images, the ratio of pulp/tooth volume could be calculated for living individuals.[5]

Swasty et al evaluated the cortical thickness, height and width with CBCT, and determined the relationship between these parameters and age. Variation in mandibular cortical bone thickness, height, width changes are age, gender and facial type dependent.[6]

More and more CBCT examinations are being performed worldwide and contain important information for the quantitative study of dental tissue. Although CBCT examinations are conducted in the first intention of making a clinical diagnosis or prognostic evaluation, they could be used as an initial database for the measurement of dental volumes and their ratios, thus furnishing preliminary evaluations and information, which could be used later as when required.[1]

Volumetric measurements are obtained by the segmentation method with a specific software package. There is no fully automatic segmentation method available as yet, but semiautomatic segmentation is possible. Currently, segmentation of a tooth is more difficult, when it is adjacent to cortical bone.[7] Future research is required to automatic segmentation and improve the signal-to-noise ratio, and the contrast. The newest CBCT operating modes and optimization of the ratio measurement software, together with increased number of samples, could bring the technique to maturity in forensic odontology research.[1]

CBCT IN SEXUAL DIMORPHISM

The identification of sex is considered to be an important step in the reconstruction of the biological profile of an unknown individual in the forensic context. The techniques used are based on assessments of the morphological characteristics of the pelvis and skull, but in some cases the basin or the pelvis is in a fragmentary state.[8] In the forensic setting, anthropologists have long used teeth as an additional tool to determine sex because of their ability to resist destruction after death. In this situation, the use of data from a specific population is important because sexual dimorphism varies among different populations.[8,9]

Sexual dimorphism is a method that has been used for many years within forensic dentistry for human identification. This method is better in adults because of the morphological influences that affect bone structure such as the hormones that control growth, bone development and developments during puberty. In contemporary populations, there is a relative scarcity of specific morphometric patterns for estimating sex from bone findings from unidentified human remains. There is basically a lack of historical evidence or documentation on the use of human skeletons available for study.[8]

Previous studies have indicated that the relative position of the inferior alveolar canal and its respective mental foramina in adults can be used to estimate sexual dimorphism and age. Arguably, these differences can be used as proposed values for forensic identification of human remains. In forensic medicine, numerous studies have used computed tomography (CT) as an auxiliary method in the discovery of unidentified bodies postmortem. Thus, several authors have reported on the important benefits of CT in assisting coroners. CBCT is the test of choice in dentistry and has the advantage of much lower cost, and smaller size of the equipment without losing reliability and accuracy of the image compared with multidetector CT (MDCT).[8]

Cone beam computed tomography has been useful to determine the characteristic positioning of the mandibular canal and the mental foramina can facilitate differentiation between the sexes, when the mandible of a missing person is found. The main advantage of CBCT over CT is that it is associated with considerably fewer metal artifacts and is thus able to localize metallic foreign objects. However, it is not a specific examination for soft tissue. Thus, CBCT provides better image quality, when metallic objects are present in the oral cavity. CBCT can assist professionals in forensic human identification, providing a fast and precise method. It also offers the possibility of using a formula that allows sex differentiation of individuals from measurements on mandibular anatomic structures.[8]

Study done by Behzad Nejat, he reliably produced CBCT-derived measurements that were comparable to data from a sex identification method on lateral cephalometric radiographs.[8,9] These were validated in Taiwanese, European, Indian adults.[9-11]

Nejat used similar protocol in Hispanic females and found that the mean and standard deviations of the cephalometric sex identification measurements in this study are comparable to those reported by Hsiao, Chang and Liu.[11] As shown by Patil, Mody Veyre-Goulet, Mercier, Robin and Guerin different ethnic populations have unique mean values for this anatomic variables.[11,12]

CBCT IN FACIAL APPROXIMATION

Nejat outlined a method to produce rapid facial approximations to aid forensic identification, while employing minimal computation or graphical complexity. The results of the facial approximation section of this study implies the ability of cephalometric measurements to create approximated soft tissue profiles from skull data alone.[10] The introduction of CBCT imaging into the orthodontic diagnostic record taking process has introduced commonality between the forensic facial reconstruction and orthodontic fields that would be required to be fully explored.

CONCLUSION

The CBCT technology enables us to envisage new research oriented toward various aspects of teeth and jaws, which could play an important role in forensic field, thanks to its broad sampling possibilities.

REFERENCES

1. Maret D, Peter OA, Dedouit F, et al. Cone-Beam Computed Tomography: a useful tool for dental age estimation? Med Hypotheses. 2011;76(5):700-2.
2. Demirjian A, Goldstein H. New systems for dental maturity based on seven and four teeth. Ann Hum Biol. 1976;3(5):411-21.
3. Saunders S, DeVito C, Herring A, et al. Accuracy trends of tooth formation age estimations for human skeletal remains. Am J Phys Anthropol. 1993;92(2):173-88.
4. Cameriere R, Ferrante L, Belcastro MG, et al. Age estimation by pulp/tooth ratio in canines by mesial and vestibular peri-apical X-rays. J Forensic Sci. 2007;52(5):1151-5.
5. Yang F, Jacobs R, Willems G. Dental age estimation through volume matching of teeth imaged by cone-beam CT. Forensic Sci Int. 2006;159 suppl 1:78-83.
6. Swasty D, Lee JS, Huang JC, et al. Anthropometric analysis of the human mandibular cortical bone as assessed by cone-beam computed tomography. J Oral Maxillofac Surg. 2009;67(3):491-500.
7. Liu Y, Olszewski R, Alexandroni ES, et al. The validity of in vivo tooth volume determinations from cone-beam computed tomography. Angle Orthod. 2010;80(1):160-6.
8. Gamba T, Alves MC, Neto FH. Analysis of sexual dimorphism by locating the mandibular canal in images of cone-beam computed tomography. JOFRI. 2014;2(2):72-76.
9. Zorba E, Moraitis K, Manolis SK. Sexual dimorphism in permanent teeth of modern Greeks, Forensic Sci Int. 2011;210 (1-3):74-81.
10. Nejat Behzad. 'A Forensic Identification Utility to Create Facial Approximations using Cone-Beam Computed Tomography of 100. Hispanic Females: A Pilot Study'. UNLV Theses/Dissertations/Professional Papers/Capstones. Paper 1763; 2012.
11. Hsiao TH, Chang HP, Liu KM. Sex determination by discriminant function analysis of lateral radiographic cephalometry. J Forensic Sci. 1996;41(5):792-5.
12. Patil KR, Mody RN. Determination of sex by discriminant function analysis and stature by regression analysis: a lateral cephalometric study. Forensic Sci Int. 2005;147(2-3): 175-80.

12 Chapter

Limitations of Cone Beam Computed Tomography

Prashant P Jaju

INTRODUCTION

Cone beam computed tomography (CBCT) has brought a paradigm shift in diagnosis and treatment in dental field. Three-dimensional (3D) imaging of CBCT surpasses the shortcomings of two-dimensional (2D) images. However, CBCT is not all inclusive technology as it suffers from some inherent limitations. While clinical applications of CBCT have expanded, current CBCT technology has limitations related to the 'cone beam' projection geometry, detector sensitivity and contrast resolution that produce images that lack the clarity and usefulness of conventional computed tomography (CT) images. The clarity of CBCT images is affected by artifacts, noise and poor soft tissue contrast.

POOR SOFT TISSUE CONTRAST

Soft tissue swellings in head and neck region, meniscal anatomy of temporomandibular joint (TMJ), vascular lesions cannot be appreciated adequately on CBCT images due to inherent poor soft tissue contrast. Three factors limit the contrast resolution of CBCT. Although scattered radiation contributes to increased image noise, it is also a significant factor in reducing the contrast of the cone beam system. In addition, the divergence of the X-ray beam over the area detector causes a pronounced heel effect. This effect produces a inhomogeneity or nonuniformity of the incident X-ray beam on the patient and resultant nonuniformity in absorption, with greater signal-to-noise ratio (noise) on the cathode side of the image relative to the anode side. Finally, numerous inherent flat panel detector-based artifacts affect its linearity or response to X-radiation. Although these conditions limit the application of current CBCT imaging to the assessment of osseous structures, several techniques and devices are currently being investigated to suppress this effect.[1]

LACK OF PRECISE HOUNSFIELD VALUES

The Hounsfield (HU) scale that is used in CT is calculated from the linear attenuation coefficient (m) value of each tissue and takes into account the linear attenuation coefficient of water. The HU is not part of the system international (SI). It is neither a SI fundamental unit nor a derived unit; rather, it is a useful practical unit that represents the relative deviation of the measured linear attenuation of a material from that of water. X-ray beams used for diagnostic radiology are not monochromatic (i.e. consisting of photons with only one energy) and are thus composed of photons with a broad spectrum of energies. This is the fundamental reason why the HU value for a tissue obtained from one CT system may not be the same as that obtained with a different CT system (or even with the same machine if different technique factors are used). The CT is inherently prone to artifacts that reduce the accuracy of HUs for measurement of physical density. The HUs derived from CBCT systems have more sources of errors than do multidetector computed tomography (MDCT) systems and greater cost constraints for correction. With more advanced CBCT software and methods, it should be possible to improve the accuracy of CBCT HU values for determining physical densities.[2]

RADIATION DOSE

Radiation dose delivered by CBCT is less compared with CT. Panoramic radiography and intraoral radiographs deliver a low dose compared with CBCT (refer Chapter 2, 'Cone Beam Computed Tomography: Physics and Artifacts'). Hence, the as low as reasonably achievable (ALARA) principle should be followed properly. Understanding the radiation dose imparted to patients with the use of CT and CBCT technologies, both of which use ionizing radiation as an important patient safety issue. Therefore, it is imperative for operators of both technologies to use specific exposure imaging protocols that provide images with sufficient image quality to answer a specific diagnostic concern with the least amount of radiation. Proper patient selection, adequately selected field of view (FOV) depending upon the indication of CBCT scan, this limitation of radiation dosage could be overcome adequately.[1]

DENTAL CARIES

Early incipient dental caries, pit and fissure caries are diagnosed adequately on intraoral radiographs rather than CBCT. At this time, the application of CBCT imaging to caries diagnosis is promising, with more research needed, especially in vivo investigations. In addition, with current technology, it is assumed that teeth with metal or even radiopaque restorations should not be considered for CBCT caries imaging, as metallic artifacts hide the carious lesions.

COST OF SCANS

Cone beam computed tomography technology is an expensive proposition. The initial investment for the dentists/oral radiologists is pretty high. With introduction of hybrid CBCT machines the cost factor is reducing significantly. In developing countries like India, where dental insurance are not available to patients, cost of CBCT scans could be possible hindrance for referring patients for scanning. But with proper indication and wealth of information provided by CBCT scans, this limitation of CBCT scan is easily overcome. This is not the limitation of CBCT technology, but lack of proper patient selection.

CONCLUSION

Future of CBCT machines will depend upon improvement in soft tissue imaging, reduction of cost and increase in the number of radiology centers having CBCT machines.

REFERENCES

1. Angelopoulos C, Scarfe WC, Farman AG. A comparison of maxillofacial CBCT and medical CT. Atlas Oral Maxillofac Surg Clin North Am. 2012;20(1):1-17.
2. Molteni R. Prospects and challenges of rendering tissue density in Hounsfield units for cone beam computed tomography. Oral Surg Oral Med Oral Pathol Oral Radiol. 2013;116(1):105-19.

Glossary

A

Abscess: A localized collection of pus within a tissue or a confined space.

Abutment: A connector placed on or built into the top of the dental implant to connect the implant to the replacement tooth or teeth.

Accessory canal: Any branch of the main pulp canal or chamber that communicates with the external surface of the root.

Accessory foramen: An orifice on the surface of a root communicating with a lateral or accessory canal.

Acute apical abscess: An inflammatory reaction to pulpal infection and necrosis characterized by rapid onset, spontaneous pain, tenderness of the tooth to pressure, pus formation and swelling of associated tissues.

ALARA: Acronym for as low as reasonably achievable. It refers to the principle that all radiation exposure, both to patients and to radiologic personnel, should be minimized in diagnostic imaging.

Alveolar process: The alveolar process (alveolar bone) is the thickened ridge of bone that contains the tooth sockets (dental alveoli) on bones and hold teeth.

Apical foramen: The main apical opening of the root canal.

Arthritis: It Greek 'arthro' means joint and 'itis' means inflammation; plural—arthritides is a form of joint disorder that involves inflammation of one or more joints.

Artifact: It can present in a variety of ways including abnormal shadow noted on a radiograph or degraded image quality and have been produced by artificial means from hardware failure, operator error and software (post-processing) artifacts.

Asymptomatic apical periodontitis: Inflammation and destruction of apical periodontium that is of pulpal origin, appears as an apical radiolucent area and does not produce clinical symptoms.

B

Beam hardening: The process of increasing the average energy level of an X-ray beam by filtering out the low-energy photons.

Bisecting angle technique: The X-ray beam is directed at a right angle to an imaginary plane that bisects the angle formed by the film and the central axis of the tooth; the film is placed as close as possible to the tooth.

Bone density (or bone mineral density): It is a medical term normally referring to the amount of mineral matter per square centimeter of bones.

Bone quality: Encompasses factors other than bone density such as skeletal size, the architecture and 3D orientation of the trabecular and matrix properties.

Buccal object rule: A method for determining the relative location of objects that are superimposed on the traditional radiograph. The rule is 'When two different radiographs are made of a pair of objects, the image of the buccal objects moves relative to the image of the lingual object in the opposite direction from which the X-ray beam is directed'.

C

CAD/CAM: It is a field of dentistry and prosthodontics using computer-aided design and computer-aided manufacturing (CAD/CAM) to improve the design and creation of dental restorations, especially dental prostheses including crowns, crown lays, veneers, inlays and onlays, fixed bridges, dental implant restorations, dentures (removable or fixed) and orthodontic appliances.

Cancellous bone: Synonymous with trabecular bone or spongy bone, is one of two types of osseous tissue that form bones. It is typically found at the ends of long bones, proximal to joints and within the interior of vertebrae. It is highly vascular and frequently contains red bone marrow, where hematopoiesis, the production of blood cells occurs. The primary anatomical and functional unit of cancellous bone is the trabecula.

Caries: A localized and progressive bacterial infection that results in the disintegration of a tooth, usually beginning with the dissolution of enamel and followed by bacterial invasion.

CEREC or Cerec (Chairside Economical Restoration of Esthetic Ceramics or Ceramic Reconstruction): It is a method of CAD/CAM dentistry developed by Mörmann W and Brandestini M at the University of Zurich in 1980 for creating dental restorations.

Cervical resorption: A type of external resorption that occurs in the coronal third of the root.

Chronic apical abscess: An inflammatory reaction to pulpal infection and necrosis characterized by gradual onset, little or no discomfort and the intermittent discharge of pus through an associated sinus tract.

Collimation: The process of restricting and confining X-ray beam to a given area.

Computed tomography: Radiography in which a three-dimensional (3D) image of a body structure is constructed by computer from a series of plane cross-sectional images made along an axis also called computed axial tomography, computerized axial tomography or computed tomography.

Cone beam computed tomography: It is a medical imaging technique consisting of X-ray computed tomography, where the X-rays are divergent, forming a cone.

Contrast: Difference in the degree of blackness between adjacent areas on a dental radiograph.

Contrast resolution: Is the ability of an imaging system to distinguish minor differences in tissue attenuation and to display them with different gray levels.

Cortical bone: Synonymous with compact bone, is one of the two types of osseous tissue that form bones. Cortical bone facilitates bone's main functions, i.e. to support the whole body, protect organs, provide levers for movement, and store and release chemical elements, mainly calcium. As its name implies, cortical bone forms the cortex or outer shell of most bones.

Crown: A replacement tooth, custom made to match the natural teeth.

Cyst: An epithelium-lined pathologic cavity that may contain fluid, semi-solid material or cellular debris; oral and perioral cysts frequently classified as odontogenic, nonodontogenic, soft tissue and pseudocysts.

D

Dehiscence: A narrow, vertical defect in the alveolar plate of bone over a root extending from the crestal area apically; usually located on the facial aspect of the alveolar process.

Density: It is the overall blackness or darkness of a dental radiograph.

Dental implant: Also known as an endosseous implant or fixture, is a surgical component that interfaces with the bone of the jaw or skull to support a dental prosthesis such as a crown, bridge, denture, facial prosthesis or to act as an orthodontic anchor.

DICOM: Digital Imaging and Communications in Medicine (DICOM) is a standard for handling, storing, printing and transmitting information in medical imaging. It includes a file format definition and a network communications protocol.

Distortion: Radiographic image distortion is a variation in the true size and shape of the object being recorded.

Dosimetry: Determination of the quantity of radiation exposure or dose.

E

Ectopic tooth: A tooth that is impacted, but does manage to erupt at an angle, rather than emerging straight out. A tooth that erupts in this manner is called ectopic, meaning that it is displaced or incorrectly positioned.

External resorption: Resorption initiated in the periodontium and initially affecting the external surfaces of a tooth; may be further classified as surface, inflammatory or replacement, or by location as cervical, lateral or apical; may or may not invade the dental pulp space.

Extrusive luxation: A partial axial displacement of the tooth from its socket.

F

Fenestration: These are isolated areas in which root is denuded of bone and root surface is covered only by periosteum and overlying gingiva is called fenestration.

Field of view (FOV): The could be defined as area of interest to be covered during the scanning procedure.

Filtration: The addition of metal sheets to a beam of X-rays for the purpose of altering the energy spectrum and thus the imaging characteristics and penetrating ability of the radiation. Filtration is generally accomplished with aluminum or copper at low to medium energy and copper or aluminum at higher energy.

There are two major variants of digital image capture devices; flat panel detectors (FPDs) and high-density line-scan solid state detectors. FPDs are further classified in to two main categories:

1. **Direct FPDs:** Amorphous selenium (a-Se) FPDs are known as 'direct' detectors because X-ray photons are converted directly into charge. The outer layer of the flat panel in this design is typically a high-voltage bias electrode. X-ray photons create electron-hole pairs in a-Se, and the transit of these electrons and holes depends on the potential of the bias voltage charge. As the holes are replaced with electrons, the resultant charge pattern in the selenium layer is read out by a TFT array, active matrix array, electrometer probes or microplasma line addressing.
2. **Indirect FPDs:** Amorphous silicon (a-Si) is the most common material of commercial FPDs. Combining a-Si detectors with a scintillator in the detector's outer layer, which is made from cesium iodide (CsI) or gadolinium oxysulfide (Gd_2O_2S), converts X-rays to light. Because of this conversion the a-Si detector is considered an indirect imaging device. The light is channeled through the a-Si photodiode layer, where it is converted to a digital output signal. The digital signal is then read out by thin film transistors (TFTs) or fiber-coupled charge-coupled devices (CCDs). The image data file is sent to a computer for display.

Flat panel detectors: These are a class of solid-state X-ray digital radiography devices similar in principle to the image sensors used in digital photography and video.

Foramen: A natural opening or passage, especially into or through a bone; also describes openings in the root structure that communicate with the dental pulp and generally contain neural, vascular and connective elements.

Furcation: In dentistry furcation defect is bone loss, usually a result of periodontal disease, affecting the base of the root trunk of a tooth, where two or more roots meet.

G

Gingiva: Consist of the mucosal tissue that lies over the mandible and maxilla inside the mouth.

H

Horizontal root fracture (oblique root fracture): Fracture due to traumatic injury confined to the root in a transverse plane separating the coronal and apical segments.

Hounsfield unit (HU): Scale is a linear transformation of the original linear attenuation coefficient measurement into one in which the radiodensity of distilled water at standard pressure and temperature (STP) is defined as zero Hounsfield units.

I

Image intensifier: The term image intensifier refers to a specific component of X-ray imaging system, which allows low intensity X-rays to be converted to a visible light output.

Image noise: Refers to the density differences in a radiographic image that are attributed to statistical fluctuations on the distribution of the X-ray photons registered by the detector.

Image quality: It is a characteristic of an image that measures the perceived image degradation (typically, compared to an ideal or perfect image).

Image reconstruction: This in computed tomography (CT) is a mathematical operation that converts attenuation values per voxel from X-ray projection data to grayscale images.

Image sensor: It is a device that converts an optical image into an electronic signal. It is used mostly in digital cameras, camera modules and other imaging devices. Early analog sensors were video camera tubes; currently used types are semiconductor CCD or active pixel sensors in complementary metal oxide semiconductor (CMOS).

Each cell of a CCD image sensor is an analog device. When light strikes the chip, it is held as a small electrical charge in each photoelectrical sensor. The charges are converted to voltage one pixel at a time as they are read from the chip. Additional circuitry in the camera converts the voltage into digital information.

A CMOS imaging chip is a type of active pixel sensor made using the CMOS semiconductor process. Extra circuitry next to each photoelectrical sensor converts the light energy to a voltage. Additional circuitry on the chip may be included to convert the voltage to digital data.

Inflammatory arthritis: It is a term used to describe a group of conditions, which affect the immune system. This means that the body's defense system starts attacking own tissues instead of germs, viruses and other foreign substances, which can cause pain, stiffness and joint damage.

Inflammatory resorption: An internal or external pathologic loss of tooth structure and possibly bone, resulting in a defect; occurs as the result of microbial infection; characterized radiographically by radiolucent areas along the root.

Internal resorption: An inflammatory process initiated within the pulp space with loss of dentin and possible invasion of the cementum.

Impacted tooth: It is one that is unable to fully erupt in its proper location because it is blocked by tissue, bone or another tooth.

Intrusive luxation: An axial displacement of the tooth into the alveolus often accompanied by comminuted apical fracture of the alveolar socket.

L

Lamina dura: The layer of compact bone forming the wall of a tooth alveolus seen in dental radiographs as a thin radiopaque line surrounding the roots of teeth; loss of continuity and changes in its width and radiopacity may indicate pathosis.

Lateral luxation: A displacement of the tooth in a direction other than axially, usually accompanied by fracture of the alveolar socket.

Luxation: Displacement of a tooth from its original position in the alveolus, without total avulsion, resulting from acute trauma.

M

Magnification: Radiographic image that appears larger than the actual size of the object it represents.

Mandible: It is the largest, strongest and lowest bone in the face. It forms the lower jaw and holds the lower teeth in place.

Maxilla: These are the two maxilla bones forming the upper jaw and palate of the mouth.

Maximum intensity projection: Picks out and projects only the voxels with maximum intensity that fall in the way of parallel rays traced from the viewpoint to the plane of projection.

Microscopic abscess: Incipient collection of pus, typically so small as to be visualized only at the light microscope level.

N

Noise: It is defined as an unwanted, randomly and/or non-randomly distributed disturbance of a signal that tends to obscure the signal's information content from the observer.

O

Orthognathic surgery: Refers to a variety of procedures designed to move the upper and/or lower jaws into a different, more appropriate position.

Osseointegration: Derives from the Greek osteon, bone and the Latin integrare, to make whole. The term refers to the direct structural and functional connection between living bone and the surface of a load-bearing artificial implant.

Osteitis: Bone inflammation involving haversian spaces, canals and their branches.

Osteoarthritis: Commonly known as wear and tear arthritis, is the most common type of arthritis. It is associated with a breakdown of cartilage in joints and can occur in almost any joint in the body. It commonly occurs in the weight-bearing joints of the hips, knees and spine.

Osteomyelitis: Inflammation of bone marrow and adjacent bone caused by an infectious organism, often the staphylococci; inflammation may remain localized or may spread throughout the bone to involve the marrow, cortex, cancellous tissue and periosteum. Chronic osteomyelitis may follow acute osteomyelitis and usually necessitates treatment with surgical and chemotherapeutic (antibiotics) intervention.

Osteoporosis: A metabolic bone disease of variable etiologies that results in a net decrease in bone mass; characterized by disproportionate osteoclastic activity in cells.

Osteotomy (ostectomy): Surgical access in bone, typically used to access root end.

P

PACS: Picture archiving and communication system (PACS) is a medical imaging technology, which provides economical storage of and convenient access to images from multiple modalities (source machine types).

Panoramic radiograph: Radiographic procedure that produces a single tomographic image of facial structures including both maxillary and mandibular arches, and their supporting structures.

Paralleling technique (long cone technique): The X-ray film is supported parallel to the long axis of the teeth and the central ray of the X-ray beam is directed at right angles to the teeth and film; to reduce geometric distortions, it is important that the X-ray source be located relatively distant from the teeth, hence the use of a long cone.

Periodontal abscess: Also termed as lateral abscess or parietal abscess, is a localized collection of pus (i.e. an abscess) within the tissues of the periodontium or an inflammatory reaction originating in the periodontium; usually characterized by rapid onset, spontaneous pain, tenderness of the tooth to pressure, pus formation and swelling; frequently caused by foreign body entrapment and often associated with a tooth with a vital pulp.

Periodontitis (pericementitis): Inflammation of the periodontium.

Periodontium: The tissues that surround and support teeth, attaching them to the alveolar bone includes bone, connective tissue, vascular and neuronal elements.

Periradicular: Surrounding the root.

Pixel: Picture element is a physical point in a raster image or the smallest addressable element in an all points addressable display device; so it is the smallest controllable element of a picture represented on the screen.

Pulp: A richly vascularized and innervated specialized connective tissue of ectomesenchymal origin; contained in the central space of a tooth, surrounded by the dentin with inductive, formative, nutritive, sensory and protective functions.

Pulp abscess: A localized collection of clinically visible pus within the pulp of the tooth; initiated by microorganisms and/or its byproducts.

R

Radiation: It is a process in which electromagnetic radiation (EMR) travel through a vacuum or through matter-containing media; the existence of a medium to propagate the waves is not required.

Radiograph: An image produced by the action of X-rays.

Radiographic techniques: Methods for making radiographic images using film and X-ray source.

Radiography: It is an imaging technique that uses electromagnetic radiation other than visible light, especially X-rays, to view the internal structure of a non-uniformly composed and opaque object (i.e. a non-transparent object of varying density and composition) such as the human body.

Radiology information system (RIS): It is a network software suite for managing medical imagery and associated data.

Radiolucency (rarefaction): An area of darkness on a radiograph indicating that an object of low density is allowing complete or partial penetration by X-rays.

Radiopacity: An area of lightness on a radiograph indicating that the density of an object is preventing penetration by X-rays.

Replacement resorption (ankylosis): A pathologic loss of cementum, dentin and periodontal ligament with subsequent replacement of such structures by bone, resulting in fusion of bone and tooth.

Resolution: Capability of X-ray to reproduce distinct outlines of an object or to reproduce the smallest details of an object on a dental radiograph.

Resorption: A condition associated with either a physiologic or a pathologic process resulting in a loss of dentin, cementum and/or bone.

Root canal: A passage or channel in the root of the tooth extending from the pulp chamber to the apical foramen; may be narrow, have lateral branches and/or exhibit irregular morphology.

Root canal system: The space containing the dental pulp inside the crown and root of a tooth.

Root fracture: Limited to fractures of root structure involving cementum, dentin and pulp.

S

Sequestrum: It is a piece of dead bone that has become separated during the process of necrosis from normal or sound bone. It is a complication (sequela) of osteomyelitis.

Sialography: It is the radiographic examination of the salivary glands. It usually involves the injection of a small amount of contrast medium into the salivary duct of a single gland, followed by routine X-ray projections.

SLOB rule: When two different radiographic angles are compared, the more lingual structure moves in the same direction as the X-ray tube head, while the more buccal object moves opposite.

Spatial resolution: It is the ability of the imaging system to distinguish small structures that lie close to one another.

Stereophotogrammetry: It is emerging as a robust non-contacting measurement technique to determine dynamic characteristics and mode shapes of non-rotating and rotating structures.

Subluxation: An abnormal loosening of the tooth in the alveolar socket without displacement.

Surgical guides: These are appliances that are computer designed and are fabricated of an acrylic resin by a process called stereolithography.

Symptomatic apical periodontitis: Inflammation usually of the apical periodontium producing clinical symptoms including a painful response to biting and/or percussion or palpation. It might or might not be associated with an apical radiolucent area.

T

Tomography: It is a process by which an image layer of the body is produced, while the images of the structures above and below the layer are made invisible by blurring.

V

Vertical root fracture: Fracture occurs most frequently in endodontically treated teeth; characterized by a crack that begins in the root and extends toward the occlusal surface, usually buccal-lingual; may be associated with an isolated periodontal defect; radiographic detection may be difficult due to superimposed obturation and restorative materials.

Volume rendering: It is a set of techniques used to display a 2D projection of a 3D discretely sampled data set, typically a 3D scalar field.

Voxel: It represents a value on a regular grid in 3D space. Voxel is a combination of 'volume' and 'pixel,' where pixel is a combination of 'picture' and 'element.'

X

X-ray: Electromagnetic radiation emitted from bombardment of a target anode with a stream of electrons from a heated cathode; passes through solid bodies, can cause destructive changes in living tissues and affects a photographic emulsion.

Index

Page numbers followed by '*f*' and '*t*' indicate figures and tables respectively.